For Kellie,
Thanks for helping women
fight the good fight.
Best,
Liz xx

Conceivability

WHAT I LEARNED
EXPLORING *the* FRONTIERS
of FERTILITY

ELIZABETH KATKIN

Simon & Schuster

NEW YORK   LONDON   TORONTO   SYDNEY   NEW DELHI

Simon & Schuster
1230 Avenue of the Americas
New York, NY 10020

Copyright © 2018 by Elizabeth Katkin

The names of some individuals in this book have been changed.

First Simon & Schuster hardcover edition June 2018

SIMON & SCHUSTER and colophon are registered trademarks of Simon & Schuster, Inc.

For information about special discounts for bulk purchases, please contact
Simon & Schuster Special Sales at 1-866-506-1949 or business@simonandschuster.com.

The Simon & Schuster Speakers Bureau can bring authors to your live event.
For more information or to book an event, contact the Simon & Schuster Speakers Bureau
at 1-866-248-3049 or visit our website at www.simonspeakers.com.

Interior design by Ruth Lee-Mui

Manufactured in the United States of America

1   3   5   7   9   10   8   6   4   2

Library of Congress Cataloging-in-Publication Data

Names: Katkin, Elizabeth L., author.
Title: Conceivability : what I learned exploring the frontiers of fertility / Elizabeth Katkin.
Description: New York : Simon & Schuster, 2018. | Includes bibliographical references and index.
Identifiers: LCCN 2017053978| ISBN 9781501142369 (hardback) | ISBN 9781501142376
(trade paperback) | ISBN 9781501142383 (ebook)
Subjects: LCSH: Katkin, Elizabeth L.,—Health | Infertility. | Infertility—Treatment. | Conception.
| Polycystic ovary syndrome—Treatment. | BISAC: BIOGRAPHY & AUTOBIOGRAPHY / Personal
Memoirs. | HEALTH & FITNESS / Pregnancy & Childbirth. | HEALTH & FITNESS / Infertility.
Classification: LCC RC889 .K358 2018 | DDC 618.1/780092 [B] —dc23
LC record available at https://lccn.loc.gov/2017053978

ISBN 978-1-5011-4236-9
ISBN 978-1-5011-4238-3 (ebook)

For Richard,
Alexandra, and William
without whom my life would be inconceivable

In Loving Memory

Dorothy Gadasin Freedman
aka GGM
A terrific woman of extraordinary strength
who waited until her ninety-seventh year for the arrival
of her youngest beloved great-grandchild

Caryn Katkin Pally
Mother, daughter, sister, wife
who believed in family
and the power of sibling love

Elizabeth and Walter Wawrzyniak
who overcame inconceivable obstacles
to raise their children with unconditional love
and instill the belief that anything was possible

Contents

    Gestational Surrogacy   115

10. When It Takes a Village: *Surrogacy and Egg Donation*   134

11. Louise's Legacy: *The Business of Baby-making*   162

12. Pricing the "Priceless": *Big Money and the Finance
    of Fertility*   178

13. The Good, the Bad, and the Eggs: *The Fundamental
    Debate About Egg Integrity*   198

14. Minding the Gaps: *Reflections on the Future of Fertility*   215

    Epilogue   235

    Afterword by Dr. Joel Batzofin   237

    Acknowledgments   241

    Notes   247

    Index   283

ななころびやおき *(Nana korobi ya oki)*
Fall down seven times, stand up eight.

Japanese proverb

If opportunity doesn't knock, build a door.

Milton Berle

Introduction

"*If* you have to write a book, why can't you write a book about recipes, like how to make cookies?" asked my then five-year-old daughter, with her impish little grin.

I scooped out the dough onto a baking sheet, smiling. "Because I want to write a book about how to make babies," I answered, "so that other parents can have wonderful babies like you and your brother."

Alexandra looked at me, her striking green eyes wide with indignation. "I am *not* a baby," she cried.

"You know what I mean," I replied. "You were a baby."

"But having babies is easy," Alexandra declared. "Everybody has babies." She twirled around on her toes, practicing to be a ballerina. "When I grow up, I am going to have a girl and a boy. An older sister and a younger brother. Sarah and Henry."

"Just like that?" I asked.

"Just like that."

I had thought so too. Like Alexandra, I used to believe I would grow up and get married and have two children, one boy and one girl, just like my parents did. Just like that.

I never thought for even a second about the possibility that it might not happen. Until the time came when I actually tried to get pregnant, my only pregnancy concern had been ensuring that it didn't happen accidentally.

I looked at my beautiful daughter practicing her ballet steps in the kitchen and, not for the first time, marveled at her very existence. If she only knew the amount of time, energy, and money—not to mention the physical and emotional ordeal—that her father and I had gone through over the last decade to create her and her brother.

I never could have imagined that my quest for children would ultimately look like this:

Seven miscarriages
Eight fresh IVF cycles
Two frozen IVF attempts
Five natural pregnancies
Four IVF pregnancies
Ten doctors (four of whom told me to give up trying)
Six countries
Two potential surrogates
Nine years
$200,000

That's my recipe. And now my husband and I have two beautiful, healthy children. One boy and one girl. Just like that.

I am an accidental fertility expert. I did not go to medical school, and did not, in my college and graduate years, prepare to devote myself to helping other women, let alone myself, get pregnant. Fertility was not something I ever thought about, until confronted with years of "trying" and the devastating pain of my first miscarriage—sadly followed by six additional miscarriages and almost a dozen failed IVF attempts. Yet I surprised even myself in my absolute, unshakable refusal to take no for an answer. In the face of overwhelming challenges, I gradually undertook my own quest to find solutions.

In so doing, I was willing to sacrifice a lot—too much, some might say, and some did. I submitted my body to punishing rounds of fertility treatments of every kind. I was willing to spend every cent of our life savings. I saw doctors at top clinics in six countries—the United States, the United Kingdom, Switzerland, Germany, the United Arab Emirates, and Russia—and educated myself on state-of-the-art Western practices, as well as ancient Eastern and traditional approaches to overcoming infertility. I tried intrauterine insemination (IUI), in vitro fertilization (IVF), intracytoplasmic sperm injection (ICSI), preimplantation genetic diagnosis (PGD), and in vitro immunoglobulin (IVIG). I worked with egg donors and surrogates, and completed an adoption home study. I drank Chinese herbal teas, served as a cushion for an uncountable number of acupuncture needles, and took a variety of homeopathic remedies and tinctures derived from Germany to the Arabian Peninsula. I wore a fertility necklace, touched a fertility stone, and sat under a fertility tree. Alternately a fan and a skeptic, and ultimately a realist, in my 3,285-day crusade to complete my family, I left no stone unturned, and I opened my mind to paths previously unknown to me.

I know I must sound like a zealot. I didn't start out that way. I was just a stubborn woman who wanted to have a baby, who wanted to understand why she was having difficulty, and who wanted to fix whatever was causing it. What was happening in my body? Why couldn't the doctors answer my questions? If there had been an explanation—a credible explanation—for what was wrong, I might have accepted it and moved on. But I had been trained as a lawyer, and I thought like one, and the reasons I was given didn't make sense to me and didn't hold up under interrogation. Didn't modern medicine have a way to fix what were described as commonplace problems?

Each problem I encountered had a simple, doctor-prescribed solution. I'd try the simple solution, and it worked. But I still didn't have a baby. We'd then discover a second problem, and I'd try a second solution, and it worked too. On and on it went. New problems, new solutions. I followed each prescription to a tee. But I still didn't have a baby. After multiple miscarriages and four years, instead of satisfactory explanations, there were only pieces of a puzzle that didn't seem to connect. So I did what lawyers do. I looked for answers in the facts.

I talked to doctors and researchers, communicated with other women with fertility issues, and read anything and everything available on the topic, whether written for medical professionals, laypeople, or patients. I transformed from an ardent believer in following doctors' orders to an active advocate for myself. Gradually, and somewhat unwittingly, I began to take over the management of my own case. Sometimes I knew as much as or more about my problems than my doctors. Instead of accepting the word of one doctor, I aggressively consulted with multiple doctors to create a more complete picture. I experimented on my own body with numerous mainstream, alternative, and complementary treatments.

In my elusive, and obsessive, quest for a baby, over the course of nine years I explored every conceivable—and inconceivable—path, including not only most forms of assisted reproduction but also third-party parenting (surrogacy and egg donation) and adoption.

When I was trying to conceive, there was plenty of material about IVF and how it works, but it was rare to find good advice on next steps when it doesn't work. And though there were books on coping with miscarriage, I couldn't find any on how not to miscarry.

Shockingly, it was not until the final stages of my journey that I learned that there were different perspectives—indeed, entirely different *philosophies*—on infertility treatment that might have shortened my journey. Doctors in other countries had varied approaches to infertility based on their markedly different perspective on egg quality—a major, if not the primary, culprit in failed pregnancies. It was also not until the end of my quest, in 2010, that I understood the extent of the differences between basic scientific research, the protocols of the majority of doctors treating infertility in the United States, and those used elsewhere around the world.

After nine years of seeking fertility advice and treatments, still trying to build our family, I sat in a spare, white medical examining room in a yellow house in the outskirts of Moscow, and was abruptly informed by a fast-talking Russian doctor that, in her view, the very treatments I had been pursuing for years as "the answer" had likely *hindered* rather than aided my chances of having a healthy baby, or any baby at all for that matter.

Fertility, like life, is complex, yet we usually consider it in the most simplistic fashion. We may not all be able to go to Harvard, or become president of the United States, but we can all grow up to have a family, can't we? In fact, from our teenaged lives onward, we are taught that we are likely to get pregnant any time we have unprotected sex, as long as we are not too old. For as we age, we are told, our chances of conceiving decrease as the forces of time take their irreversible toll on our eggs.

Doggedly trying to fulfill my desire to become a mother, I pursued methods consistent with this narrative. But in that clinic in Moscow, I learned that the narrative was at best oversimplified and not necessarily in line with the evolving science relating to egg and embryo quality. The doctors in Russia raised new, fundamental questions. What if, contrary to common Western medical belief, egg quality *can* be improved over time, not just left to degrade? What if our immediate environment affects the chromosomal makeup of our unborn children? What if large doses of fertility drugs, as commonly prescribed by most American fertility clinics, are *not* the most effective path for some of the fertility challenged among us?

Eventually, my husband and I found our way to having two biological children—the first conceived in New York following a traditional Anglo-American IVF protocol under the care of a South African–born doctor, the second conceived in Russia using a lower-dosage protocol after US specialists told me to give up trying—both born in the United Kingdom. Based on the knowledge I acquired along the way, I became convinced that it should not have taken so long.

The infertility problem in America—and much of the Western world—is large and growing. In 2016, fertility rates in the United States reached an all-time low.[1]

Every year, more than seven million women in the United States alone experience trouble conceiving or maintaining a pregnancy; that's more than one in eight women and one in six married couples.[2] While this book stems from and reflects my own quest for motherhood, the challenges and obstacles I faced are shared by so many. More than *one million* women a year in the United States alone seek medical help for their infertility, and at least 10 percent of all American women seek help at some point in their lives.[3] In this book, I will introduce you to some of them.

The insatiable drive to have a baby, paired with the steady rise in infertility, has set the stage for explosive growth in the fertility "industry," which is, as the word implies, as much a commercial endeavor as it is a medical practice. In addition to its stated objective of helping patients have babies, it is a business strongly influenced by other factors—clinic success rates, profits, and "the tyranny of the orthodoxy" among them. It is also a business in which the "customers," desperate for a baby and largely lacking a medical background, tend to optimistically and unquestioningly follow the advice of their doctors or fertility clinics—if they can afford such help or are fortunate enough to have insurance coverage for it.

My journey raised many questions. Why is IVF in America the most expensive in the world, but not necessarily the most successful? How do doctors and clinics define "success," and how can one be sure that the success rates clinics report are accurate (and comparable)? What are clinics in Russia and Israel and other countries with higher success rates doing right that many clinics in the United States and the United

Kingdom are not? Why do many, if not most, US clinics prescribe higher levels of drugs for longer periods of time than low-dosage protocols used successfully in many other countries? Why are the "ethics" involved in reproductive technology so inconsistent (at best) and ignored (at worst)? What are the health risks of the various treatments, and, underlying all these questions, why are key aspects of fertility treatment unregulated in the United States? Finally, and perhaps most critically to evaluating paths to success, is egg quality influenced, for better or worse, by external factors, and if so, what can be done about it?

They were questions without easy answers. So I set out to answer them. Initially driven by the desire to discover the solution to my own fertility issues, I am now driven by a desire to share what I learned with others struggling to have their own children, and anyone else interested in understanding and navigating this challenging landscape.

I cannot pretend to know the solution to everyone's infertility problems. But I have learned how to ask the right questions. I have learned that there are varied perspectives. I have learned that the American way is not the only—or necessarily the best—way for all women. I have learned that individuals need to become their own medical advocates and push for the very best care available to them. I have gained a wealth of knowledge about the medical, legal, financial, and emotional terrain involved in trying to have a child, both domestically and internationally. The information and insights I have obtained may help others who do not have the luxury to spend so much time and money searching the world for best practices. Because I was fortunate enough to be able to seek advice from a wide variety of medical professionals around the globe, I have benefited from state-of-the-art knowledge that might help others have a child more easily—specifically, *evolving knowledge about the ability to improve egg quality, therefore radically improving the odds of healthy embryos and healthy babies.*

Ever since I had my children, I have been helping friends, and friends of friends, and cousins of friends all over the world to conceive and carry their babies. My husband calls it my "side practice." Playing a role in any way toward helping would-be parents bring a baby into this world is the most gratifying thing I've ever done. Strikingly, these families did not need vast resources or an ability to travel the globe to benefit from my knowledge. To the contrary, many of the families I have advised have never left their hometown, and others have traveled to places in which treatment is in fact significantly cheaper than in the United States.

At its core, *Conceivability* represents a mind-set: a willingness to re-examine the fundamentals of our fertility practice; an ability to imagine differing conceptions of conception, whether in diagnosis, treatment, or general perspective; an acceptance of the idea that there are ways of bringing a child into the world other than the fairy-tale path we all imagine. For I have learned that options nearly always exist, and the dream of having a family should not be left on the doorstep of a fertility clinic.

There are many women and couples who walk on this journey. I wrote this book to let them know their experience is not isolated, and they are not alone.

Houston, we have a problem.

Apollo 13

From Here to Infertility

Frontline Infertility Treatments

*W*hen Richard and I got married, I was thirty and he was thirty-five. We are both big planners, and along with organizing our wedding and honeymoon, thinking about where we wanted to live now and in the future, and picking out colors for our new house, we had negotiated the kid thing at length well before the wedding. Two kids, not right away, but not too delayed either. I imagined we'd be a foursome by the time I was thirty-five, or shortly thereafter. I was a lawyer, working for the Washington, DC, office of a big Wall Street firm. Richard was a fund manager for an emerging-markets private-equity firm. We both worked a lot, traveled a lot, and had more than our fair share of fun. It was important to us that we have plenty of adventures together before our two kids arrived.

Eighteen months later, weary of the corporate-law grind and

encouraged by Richard, I left my law firm for a job at a start-up in Silicon Valley. So what if it required me to commute regularly from DC to California? It was the year 2000, the start-up world was exploding, and I had the energy and drive. I threw myself into preparations for my new life as a West Coast entrepreneur. Before my first trip to Mountain View, California, I was so busy agonizing over what clothes to pack that I forgot to pack my birth control pills. When I discovered them missing, I ran through my options. I wouldn't have time to get them before going to the new office in the morning. Could Richard overnight them to me? Could my doctor call in a prescription to a nearby CVS? Or . . . Wait a minute. We'd been married for a year and a half. Maybe I'd just stop taking the Pill altogether. The thought was a strange relief.

I called Richard, nervous and excited. Was he ready for a baby?

No, it turned out he was not ready for a baby. Like me, he still lived in a universe in which as soon as a healthy not-too-old woman goes off the Pill, she gets pregnant. He needed time to prepare. "Just a few more months?" he asked. I sighed, made a frantic call to a doctor cousin who faxed off a Pill prescription, and dashed to the pharmacy before it closed. *It's OK*, I consoled myself. I could use a few more months too.

As agreed, that June I stopped the Pill. When I tossed the empty pack, I thought to myself that with a little luck, I would be pregnant by the end of the year.

But things didn't go according to plan. Time passed, yet my period never returned. Month after month: nothing. I grew more agitated by the day, increasingly believing in my gut that something was terribly wrong yet not quite ready to confront it. Work was very stressful, and I buried myself in my new job.

No woman wants to believe that she has a fertility problem. And no one wants to go to that first appointment to find out. Although it should have been pretty clear that I needed an appointment—given that nearly six months after going off the Pill I was not yet ovulating, making it impossible to conceive—I still didn't make my first appointment with a gynecologist until I felt pushed. By my mother, of course. Richard and

I were due to fly to my parents' home on Long Island for Thanksgiving. My not-so-subtle mother had been dropping lots of hints about grand-children, and I hadn't had the heart to tell her that we were actually trying—or more accurately, trying to be trying. But now I wanted to have something to share with my parents when we saw them.

Although it might seem surprising, my conversations with dozens of women revealed that they too held off seeing a doctor. Many dragged their heels before going to a specialist, or even their own gynecologist, and the overwhelming majority did not commit a great deal of time or effort to choosing a fertility clinic—at least their first fertility clinic. When women or couples are ready to seek help, they often choose a doctor or clinic that was referred to them, or that was convenient, or that they have heard of, and they rarely do much digging into things like success rates. Fortunately, in the initial stages at least, the front line in fertility treatment should be fairly standard from clinic to clinic and country to country.

A first visit to a fertility clinic typically involves an exploration of a woman's cycle and health history, as well as at least a discussion of po-tential male issues. The initial task is diagnosis—or at least attempting a diagnosis. Is the woman ovulating? Are her tubes blocked? Does she have endometriosis? Are polycystic ovaries or polycystic ovarian syn-drome a concern? Does the man have sperm issues? Inadequate sperm count? Low motility (slow swimmers)? Poor morphology (form)? Are any of these identifiable issues possibly masking another issue? In assess-ing a woman's odds of conception, doctors will invariably try to assess both egg quality and egg quantity.

My first visit, unfortunately, did not follow this pattern. I began by seeing a recommended ob-gyn in Washington, DC, not dreaming that I needed a fertility clinic. I quickly received my unwelcome first clue that becoming parents was not going to be quite as simple for us as Richard and I had anticipated. Near the end of a brief conversation with the doctor, she told me that I had a condition called polycystic ovarian syn-drome (PCOS), a syndrome experienced by an estimated five million women in America (5 to 10 percent of all women of childbearing age), and one of the leading causes of infertility.

I was truly shocked by the diagnosis. There was nothing in my family history, and nothing in Richard's either, that had caused us concern about getting pregnant. Delivering the news of my diagnosis, the somewhat lethargic gynecologist blithely informed me that it was normal to go a while without a period after coming off birth control pills.

"Six months?" I asked.

"Sure. It's the polycystic ovarian syndrome. It's common," she said, thrusting a pamphlet into my hands. "Read this. It's no problem. Take Clomid, it makes you ovulate, and you can still conceive naturally."

I had a *syndrome*? "Can you tell me a little more about it?" I asked, my heart beating just a bit faster.

"Read the pamphlet," she shot back, her disorderly salt-and-pepper curls obscuring her face.

"Side effects?"

She headed for the door. "Headaches, nausea." Just as she pulled the door open for me, she added, "Take Advil."

I took the pamphlet and prescription from her hands. Clomiphene citrate, or Clomid, 50 mg taken daily, days five through nine of my (theoretical) cycle. It would assist my body with ovulation, and presumably therefore conception. I had no reason not to believe her. I was accustomed to a world in which medicine could fix many problems, even my mother's life-threatening leukemia several years earlier.

Off I went, home for Thanksgiving turkey with my polycystic ovaries, a synthetic hormone to kick-start the process by inducing a period, 50 mg tablets of Clomid, and a bottle of Advil. My head was spinning with the diagnosis, but I decided I would wait until after Thanksgiving dinner to mention our new problem to my parents. I wanted to eat my turkey and stuffing in peace. But no sooner had I taken off my coat than my mother asked me hopefully, "Any news?"

My mom is an academic, as is my dad. And my brother. And my

sister-in-law. No major obstacle or decision in our lives escapes mention without being examined and discussed in minute detail. I had no choice but to tell them about my difficulties and try to field their questions.

"What exactly is polycystic ovarian syndrome?" asked my dad.

Uncharacteristically, I had no real response.

"How does the Clomid work?" asked my mom.

Again, no good answer. I shoveled turkey into my mouth in an unnatural silence.

Those who know me know that I am rarely at a loss for words, and I am usually quick to search for answers. But the doctor had been so dismissive, treating my problem as a triviality, and it wasn't clear to me what to do or where to go next.

The reality is that I didn't probe too deeply when I was diagnosed, or for a long time after. And I have discovered that I am not alone in this passivity. Looking back, I realize that I was just happy to have an answer. The doctor told me I had a problem, and that Clomid was the answer. If I just took Clomid, I would ovulate, and then I would become pregnant. Who wouldn't want to believe that?

Had I done any research then, I'd have learned that Clomid, often the first line of attack in the war against infertility and taken by countless women in America, yields somewhat controversial results.

At first, the Clomid wasn't so bad for me. I didn't have painful headaches, as my doctor warned I might, but I also didn't ovulate. I experienced insomnia and mood swings but, for the most part, life went on. I had other things, for better or worse, to think about. The Internet bubble was bursting, along with company valuations and opportunities for fund-raising. What had started as a challenging but electrifying job in Silicon Valley had turned on its head. Deciding that the hours, travel, and stress could not be helping my poor little eggs to ovulate, and amid a tumultuous shake-up at the firm, I quit. Maybe now I would get my period.

But it was not to be. Three months after my first visit, I was back in the doctor's office. This time, it took two hours of waiting-room time for her to see me. When else would I have a chance to read *People*, *Cosmopolitan*, and *AARP The Magazine* all in one sitting?

"Still no period?" the ob-gyn asked, in her signature irritated voice. Still no period.

"Don't worry. We'll double the dose. Take one hundred milligrams. Should do the trick." She wrote up the prescription for Clomid in chicken scrawl and handed it to me. "If it doesn't work after two cycles, we'll go up to one hundred and fifty milligrams." And then she was gone. I was in the office for about three minutes. The waiting-time-to-visit-time ratio was an all-time personal record.

At 100 mg, my head hurt. It was harder and harder to sleep through the night. I snapped at my husband. And still no period.

About three months later, now nearly a year since we began trying for a baby, my dosage was increased again to 150 mg, this time prescribed by phone. I didn't know then that a third of women with polycystic ovaries—which often occur together with irregular periods—are actually resistant to Clomid, a fact my doctor either didn't know or neglected to tell me. Head throbbing, and seeing no progress, I started looking for a fertility specialist.

Clomid

The number one response to egg, ovulatory, or unexplained fertility problems is to prescribe clomiphene citrate, commonly known as Clomid. Taken orally in the early stages of each cycle, the drug is intended to assist a woman's body with ovulation, and presumably therefore conception, by stimulating the ovaries to release eggs. The most widely used of fertility drugs, Clomid has been on the front line of fertility treatment for more than fifty years and is now a major player in the multibillion-dollar fertility-drug industry.

Perhaps not surprisingly, the business of selling hormonal treatments has existed almost as long as the discovery of hormones. In the

early 1900s, a group of British researchers labeled the mysterious se-
cretions that seemed to affect human behavior "hormones" and began
to experiment with ways in which they could be transferred from one
person to another; for example, using testosterone from a fertile male
to help an infertile one.[1] These processes evolved over time, making a
critically important leap from the exceedingly difficult task of extracting existing hormones—from people, cows' ovaries, bulls' testicles—
to creating synthetic ones. A major fertility breakthrough occurred
unexpectedly in the 1960s when researchers studying clomiphene citrate as a potential oral contraceptive discovered that, to the contrary, it
induced ovulation and increased the chances of pregnancy.

Although attempts to control fertility are likely as old as childbirth itself, what was new about Clomid was its method of control: it
was the world's first successful synthetic hormone. Approved by the
Food and Drug Administration (FDA) in 1967, fittingly at about the
same time that birth control pills first burst onto the scene, Clomid
provided the sense that women now were liberated to choose when
they wanted to start their families. They could use birth control pills
to prevent unwanted pregnancy, and then, when they were ready for a
family, take Clomid to help stimulate the body. Compared to the previous options of an invasive surgical procedure with questionable efficacy or lifelong infertility, the orally administered clomiphene citrate
was revolutionary.

With the advent of Clomid, the modern-day fertility industry was
born. By 1970, demand for Clomid was so great that one doctor in
Los Angeles reported, "We don't have a vial in the house."[2] From its
explosive beginnings, Clomid has achieved pride of place over the last
fifty-plus years as the knee-jerk prescription doctors write when confronted with a woman trying to get pregnant. Yet unlike with other
fertility treatments, the underwhelming pregnancy rates (approximately 10 percent pregnancy rate per cycle) with Clomid have in fact
varied little over time,[3] while questions about its detrimental impacts
have only grown, in light of controversial studies—with conflicting

results—examining its possible links to cancer, increased incidence of miscarriage, and birth defects.

Clomid works by blocking the effects of estrogen in a woman's body, essentially preventing the estrogen from binding to its target on the egg cell. This blocking effect tricks the body into producing greater levels of the two other hormones that are essential to ovulation: follicle stimulating hormone (FSH), which causes the eggs in the ovaries to ripen, preparing for release; and luteinizing hormone (LH), which triggers the release of one or more mature eggs from the follicle. The potential side effects of these hormonal changes, however, include decreased cervical mucus and thinning of the endometrial lining, both critical elements to a successful and healthy conception and implantation.

And that's not all. Less important, but truly uncomfortable side effects include blurred vision, headaches, hot flashes, mood swings, abdominal pain, weight gain, insomnia, and nausea. Some women find the side effects so challenging that they opt to quit. The actress Helena Bonham Carter, who publicly revealed her and her husband's struggle to have their second child, cautioned of Clomid, "I had a terrible reaction to it. . . . It stressed me out beyond belief. Hormonally, I was all over the shop, and I got really low emotionally."[4] After quitting the tablets, she joined the "Clomid Club" of disbelievers.

"The Clomid wreaks havoc on some women, particularly those who tend toward depression. . . . It seems especially detrimental to women over forty or those who have low ovarian reserve, since it rarely results in the maturation of more than one follicle for them," says Jane Gregorie, owner and clinic director of Acupuncture Denver, who often treats women for the side effects of Clomid, which run the gamut from mood swings and depression to headaches and blurred vision, and perhaps most frustratingly, the thinning endometrial linings that present an additional challenge to pregnancy.

"It made me batshit crazy," Anna told me over coffee at our first meeting, and, adding insult to injury, "it didn't work." Now happily the mother of a healthy toddler, Anna battled infertility for more than three years. Although her problems were largely immunological, her journey, characteristically, began with Clomid. A social worker who counsels teens, Anna "was surrounded by people who had sex once and got pregnant." The Clomid certainly wasn't helping her cope.

Rose, a teacher in her midthirties, had a similar reaction. "I heard the drugs were going to make me a little weird, but my doctor said no, they wouldn't," she told me. Her fears were confirmed, however, after a couple of months of taking the pills. "I had the hardest emotional time on Clomid. I felt angry. I had temper tantrums. I was afraid it would lead to divorce."

While most fertility patients are only concerned with whether Clomid will work, there is also reason to worry about it working too much. Doctors don't always inform patients that when it works "too well," Clomid leads to overstimulation of the ovaries, resulting in a range of problems, from the benign "complication" of twins—occurring 8 to 10 percent of the time[5]—to the rather more threatening problems of quintuplets or ovarian hyperstimulation syndrome (OHSS), a condition in which a woman's ovaries swell, causing severe abdominal bloating.[6]

Its hormonal effects are not lost on those outside the fertility world too. Clomid, which enhances the body's natural production of progesterone and also conveniently masks steroids on drug tests, is included on the World Anti-Doping Agency list of doping agents in sports. In 2003, the celebrated baseball player Jason Giambi testified to a grand jury that he had taken steroids.[7] Included in his cocktail was a white pill that he said might have been Clomid, which some medical experts believe may have exacerbated Giambi's pituitary tumor a year later.

My doctor's belief that Clomid would stimulate my ovulation was reasonable. The majority of women who take Clomid do in fact ovulate. Yet this statistic can be misleading. In fact, while up to 60 to 80 percent of women ovulate in response to Clomid, only 15 to 20 percent of women with an irregular or nonexistent cycle actually *conceive* in a given cycle.[8] And while Clomid is prescribed routinely for women with "unexplained infertility," there is surprisingly little evidence that it really helps them—data reported by top fertility clinics, such as Shady Grove Fertility in Maryland, reveal that using Clomid for anything other than ovulatory irregularities results in a less than 10 percent pregnancy rate per cycle, even when combined with artificial insemination.[9] A Cochrane meta-analysis of seven randomized controlled studies showed that in the case of women with unexplained infertility, taking Clomid, whether alone or in conjunction with artificial insemination, had no statistical impact on pregnancy rates or live birth rates.[10] This may be in part due to some of the side effects of Clomid, which are not only unpleasant but may actually decrease the odds of getting pregnant.

Polycystic Ovaries and Polycystic Ovarian Syndrome (PCOS)

One in ten women of childbearing age in America has PCOS.[11] That's approximately five million women.[12] Though common, polycystic ovaries present a great challenge to fertility. In essence, the ovaries with the cysts do not possess all the hormones needed for an egg to fully mature. In a normal ovary, follicles (little balloon-like sacs that hold and nurture the eggs) grow and fill up with nourishing fluid. One follicle becomes the dominant follicle that, upon ovulation, bursts like an over-stuffed balloon, releasing a mature egg into the womb. With polycystic ovaries, however, the follicles start to fill up with fluid as they normally would, but due to insufficient hormones, no dominant follicle develops or pops; rather, the follicles slowly shrink, like balloons losing their air. They remain in the ovaries, some calcifying into cysts. Over time, the number of cysts may increase, causing even greater challenges to ovulation and conception.

Some women with polycystic ovaries experience other changes caused by their hormone imbalance, resulting in a syndrome known as polycystic ovarian syndrome, or PCOS. Acne, weight gain and trouble losing weight, excessive hair growth, depression, and infertility are signs of PCOS. Yet what woman hasn't experienced at least one or two of these issues in the past? It is precisely because of the vagueness of these seemingly unrelated symptoms, and for many, a lack of discomfort, that the most common hormonal disorder among women of reproductive age often goes undiagnosed. I probably had my polycystic ovaries for years and had absolutely no idea until I tried to get pregnant. In my teen years, I experienced an inexplicable weight gain that in retrospect was likely linked to my PCOS, but no one suspected this, or even raised the possibility, at the time.

The idea behind using Clomid to battle PCOS is simple: the suppression of estrogen is intended to force the struggling body to ovulate by artificially stimulating the necessary hormone production. However, despite its promise in theory, it is now known that Clomid is not the magic solution many hope it to be. In addition to the many women who fail to ovulate with Clomid, many others who do ovulate fail to conceive, likely because of poor egg quality—another challenge I, like a great many women with PCOS, later faced.

Fortunately, women with PCOS facing the challenge of trying to conceive now have another potential option to pursue: a drug called letrozole. Letrozole, an aromatase inhibitor approved by the FDA for the treatment of breast cancer, seeks to achieve the same goal as Clomid—stimulating ovulation—through a different physiological mechanism. Letrozole blocks the production of estrogen, as opposed to preventing the estrogen from binding to the egg cell, as Clomid does.[13] A study of 750 women, one of the largest to date examining infertility in women with PCOS, found letrozole to be more effective than Clomid, resulting in higher rates of ovulation, conception, pregnancy, and live birth rates.[14] Women assigned to take letrozole experienced an ovulation rate of 61.7 percent and a live birth rate of 27.5 percent, as compared with 48.3 percent and 19.1 percent, respectively, for the Clomid group. Although some experts urge caution, wanting to see more safety data on letrozole,[15] Dr. Richard Legro, the lead author of the study, said that

the researchers were "extremely encouraged that letrozole could provide a new, oral, first line therapy for this common disorder . . . with a
much lower risk of multiple pregnancy."[16]

Teen weight gain aside, I luckily suffered almost none of the other
side effects of the syndrome—except the most emotionally painful effect: the cysts prevented me from ovulating, making it impossible to
conceive without intervention.

The nursery is the room I've been longing for....

Clara Andrews Williams,

The House That Glue Built

Finding the Yellow Brick Road

Navigating the Fertility Labyrinth

While taking the 150 mg of Clomid, I started polling nearly every female friend and acquaintance I had in Washington, DC, asking for recommendations for a fertility specialist.

"Dr. Sacks," said Cori.

"Preston Sacks," said Katherine.

"I don't like my doctor," said Melissa, "but I hear someone called Dr. Sacks is supposed to be great."

Dr. Sacks! Was there only one good fertility doctor in all of Washington, DC? It seemed that way. When I called to make an appointment, the first available date was more than three months away. It felt like an eternity.

In the meantime, to my surprise and relief, I discovered that I was not alone with my fertility concerns. My friend Cori, from law school, provided not only a sympathetic ear but also a Clearblue Fertility Monitor. The Baby Computer, as we affectionately called it, goes far beyond a typical drugstore ovulation predictor kit. Rather than peeing on a stick for a few days to find out the one magic day that a woman might ovulate, the Baby Computer measures urine samples for many days of the cycle, indicating days of high fertility as well as two days of peak fertility, rendering a much broader window in which to potentially conceive.

My daily routine of peeing on a stick and taking the Clomid kept me busy while waiting for Dr. Sacks. It was beginning to consume more and more of my time and energy. Little did I know that it was just the beginning, that I soon would be fighting the fight of my life, encountering and surmounting obstacle after obstacle.

I realize now that at the start of my journey I had so little knowledge of not only the medical miracle of getting pregnant but also of the vast universe of fertility options that I was, without really knowing it, beginning to confront. Back then, as I followed my doctor's advice blindly, and went from one failed course of action to another, I never fully understood why certain choices were being made. It would have been helpful to have known from the start why and how the treatment progresses from one stage to the next.

In stark contrast to the notion of a baby made by nothing but one man, one woman, and pure love, evolution along the assisted-fertility spectrum is progressively less starry-eyed—and significantly more convoluted. Treatment options fall broadly into five, often overlapping, categories: *non-invasive* (Clomid and superovulatory drugs); *complementary and alternative therapies* (traditional Chinese medicine, acupuncture, nutrition, yoga); *minimally invasive* (intrauterine insemination, or IUI, also known as artificial insemination); *invasive assisted reproductive technology* (in vitro fertilization, or IVF, and its variations); and *third-party parenting* (sperm donation, egg donation, surrogacy).

During the course of my journey, I had an opportunity to explore nearly every option.

The First Visit with the Specialist

Going to the initial visit with the fertility specialist already somewhat knowledgeable about the treatment options is a good way to start. First, the task is to determine the specific nature of particular problems. For men, this consists of determining sperm quality and quantity. For women, the process is more complex, and it begins with analyzing the reproductive organs and assessing hormone levels. During the "get to know you" phase of what may turn into a very long-term relationship, in addition to taking a detailed patient history, a good fertility doctor should conduct a physical exam, including a pelvic ultrasound, and blood tests. The ultrasound may reveal abnormalities in the uterus, fallopian tubes, or ovaries, and it might also shed light on ovarian reserve (essentially, egg quantity) through measurement of the number of *antral follicles*. Antral follicles are tiny follicles in the ovaries, each of which contains an immature egg that can potentially develop and be ovulated in the future. It is believed that higher numbers of follicles will translate into higher numbers of eggs, rendering more chances of conception.

Blood tests to assess hormone levels can further help to get a sense of egg quantity and other ovulatory problems. Many doctors will want to start by analyzing levels of five hormones: FSH (follicle stimulating hormone), LH (luteinizing hormone), E2 (estradiol), AMH (anti-Mullerian hormone), and progesterone. Additional hormones, including prolactin (high levels of which may suppress the growth of egg follicles), testosterone (high levels likely indicate polycystic ovaries), and thyroid hormones (imbalances can result in ovulatory problems), may also be tested when there is reason to believe that they might come into play.

While I know this sounds like a lot to take on board, there are two main hormones believed to be the culprit in many cases of the fertility challenged: FSH and AMH. Although LH, E2, and progesterone are useful in detecting the health and regularity of a woman's cycle—whether a woman is ovulating, if the timing is correct, and if normal amounts of hormones were secreted in the process—doctors have historically turned to FSH levels, and are increasingly focusing on AMH levels, to determine whether a woman has a low ovarian reserve, meaning essentially that she has fewer eggs and presumably fewer chances to create a baby.

FSH is one of the primary hormones involved in a natural menstrual cycle as well as in drug-induced stimulation of the ovaries. It is the main hormone promoting the production of mature eggs in the ovaries, essentially providing the fuel for each egg inside its tiny follicle to start its development. In women with large supplies of eggs, it doesn't take much FSH to trigger the growth process. In women with fewer eggs, however, it takes a lot more FSH to stimulate an egg to grow, and the body will keep producing FSH until it gets one going. Testing a woman at the beginning of her menstrual cycle, typically on day two, three, or four of the cycle, gives an indication of how hard her body needs to work to produce an egg capable of ovulation. High levels of FSH indicate that a woman likely has a low ovarian reserve; in other words, not so many eggs left.

But high FSH levels are not always the harbinger of doom that many doctors and patients assume. For starters, FSH levels can be hard to interpret accurately for a number of reasons. First, they fluctuate. Second, they are measured by different diagnostic tests produced by different labs, resulting in a variety of "normal" ranges, making it difficult in certain cases to determine if a result is too high. Further, as noted by the respected fertility clinic Advanced Fertility Center of Chicago, while high baseline FSH "tends to be very predictive of low egg quantity, a normal result does not mean that the egg quantity is good."[1]

And while it flies in the face of conventional wisdom, the reverse can be true as well. Ilona, a thirty-eight-year-old African-American woman in Denver, was told that her odds of conception were very low due to her FSH level of 18 (on a scale in which less than 9 is considered normal, 9 to 11 is fair, 11 to 15 indicates a reduced ovarian reserve,

15 to 20 is a marked reduction, and more than 20 is a no go). After lowering her FSH to 14 following three months of acupuncture and traditional Chinese medicine (TCM), Ilona got pregnant naturally and gave birth to a healthy baby girl. Mary, a thirty-five-year-old with an FSH of 21.5 (a clear no go in the clinic's eyes) similarly had a healthy baby, naturally conceived after a few months of TCM and acupuncture. And Marcy, with a poor-looking FSH level of 17.6, eventually got her FSH down to 9.7, below the critical number of 10, which was the bright-line test her insurance company used to determine whether to cover her treatment. Ironically, she didn't require the expensive IVF she was so desperate for Aetna to cover, as Marcy too became pregnant the old-fashioned way.

Interestingly, while FSH is widely used to measure egg *quantity*, recent research indicates that it may be a strong indicator of egg *quality* as well. Whereas traditional thinking holds that FSH levels do not affect the chromosomal makeup of the eggs they are stimulating into ovulation, new studies suggest that high FSH levels correlate with, and may in fact cause chromosomal abnormalities in developing eggs. Studies in mice have shown that when FSH levels decrease, chromosomal abnormalities also decrease. Although similar studies with humans are in their very early days, there are promising initial results of women lowering their FSH levels and producing higher numbers of chromosomally normal, healthy eggs. FSH levels are not necessarily static, and women like Ilona and Marcy have both successfully lowered their FSH, relying on acupuncture, TCM, and supplements, and gotten pregnant.

Over the last five years, fertility clinics have increasingly turned toward testing AMH levels in addition to, or in some cases, instead of, FSH as the gold standard in predicting ovarian reserves, and assessing AMH is now a routine part of the initial fertility evaluation in many clinics. AMH is a hormone that is released during the growth of the antral follicles (those tiny follicles that each contain a developing egg). As a result, AMH levels correlate with the number of active antral follicles present; the higher the antral follicle count, the higher the AMH levels. Early studies are starting to show that it may be more accurate than FSH, due in part to the fact that AMH does not fluctuate significantly throughout the cycle as do FSH and other hormones, which also, conveniently, enables testing on any day of a woman's cycle, as opposed to during a limited window.[2] However, as a relatively new blood test, interpretation can be somewhat tricky as baseline "normal" levels (generally from 1.0 or 1.5 to 4.0) are not yet standardized and agreed on by all experts.[3]

Another reason the level of AMH may be more accurate is that it reflects the number of *active* follicles in the ovaries—those follicles that are growing and have a developing egg inside. While not believed to be indicative of egg quality, AMH levels can shed light on the size of the remaining egg supply. This distinction has important implications for treatment, for although women with low numbers of eggs are not likely to be good candidates for traditional IVF, it does not necessarily mean that they do not have good-quality eggs.

As with FSH, examples abound of women with alarmingly low AMH levels who have gone on to conceive healthy babies. Marcy, for example, was first told that her AMH was undetectable, and later told that it was .01, on a scale where 1.5 to 4.0 is considered normal and below 1.0 is considered worryingly low. She went on to conceive, without IVF. Ilona, similarly, had an AMH that was at first undetectable, and eventually rose to .5 and was discouraged from pursuing fertility treatments with her own eggs, yet she too conceived naturally. And Julia, a thirty-two-year-old woman with microscopic levels of AMH (.03), conceived and gave birth to a bouncing baby boy without assisted reproductive technology.

And then, of course, there are plenty of cases like mine. Normal FSH, LH, and E2. Normal thyroid. Normal insulin. But no baby.

So, while a patient can and should expect doctors to test hormone levels on that first visit, it is worth bearing in mind that they do not always provide definitive answers in and of themselves.

An Infertility Road Map?

While it would certainly be nice if all the testing I just described led to clear instructions, like those generated in mere seconds by the GPS in your phone or car, unfortunately, finding one's way through the maze of infertility treatments more closely resembles navigating through the woods with a compass.

In certain cases, the path will be clear. Many people facing infertility, for example, discover quickly that they have an identifiable issue, such as blocked tubes, or a low sperm count, which leads them down a specific treatment path. A woman with blocked tubes, for example, will be directed straight to IVF (which, by inserting the fertilized egg directly into the uterus, bypasses the need for the egg to travel through the fallopian tubes), while a man with a low sperm count is likely to be encouraged to undergo intracytoplasmic sperm injection (ICSI), a procedure that entails injecting the sperm directly into the egg, rather than taking the chance that the sperm and egg will find each other as nature intended.

When the panoply of clearly identifiable problems is eliminated, however, one enters the rabbit hole of "unexplained infertility," a world in which the culprit in the failure to conceive is generally assumed to be irreversibly poor egg quality, often coupled with irregular ovulation, or egg quantity—and frequently blamed on age. Yet contrary to conventional wisdom, research now shows that not all unexplained infertility is in fact due to advancing years.

The treatment of unexplained fertility is anything but straightforward. It requires a trial-and-error approach—channeling a bit of Sherlock Holmes, a touch of Dr. Watson, and a healthy dose of Monty Python in the search for the Holy Grail of eggs capable of fertilization. It also requires tenacity on the parts of both doctor and patient. A woman who finds herself entering this rabbit hole would be wise to put a lot of thought and research into the choice of treatment clinic, as they will vary in their approach, knowledge of cutting edge protocols, and success rates over time. Yet, ironically, the vast majority of doctors start the process in the exact same way: they prescribe Clomid. And if that fails, next in the noninvasive chain often comes superovulatory drugs.

Superovulatory Drugs

When ready to move on from Clomid, or perhaps now letrozole, each intended to stimulate one or two eggs to ovulate, many doctors and patients turn to superovulatory drugs, known as gonadotropins (which contain FSH, LH, or both), which aim to stimulate the production of multiple eggs. Unlike Clomid and letrozole, almost all gonadotropins, sold under the brand names Gonal-f, Puregon, Follistim, Menopur, Menogon, and many others, are injectables. Getting the balance right here is key. The goal is to help produce one or two high-quality eggs, but not too many, for if the injectables work too well, having unprotected sex (or, of course, any insemination) bears a great risk of pregnancy with multiples, enhancing risk for the mother and babies. My conversations with several women who took gonadotropins illustrate the unpredictable course that may follow when stimulating many eggs.

When Jessica and Ethan began their infertility treatment in North Carolina, their doctor suggested superovulatory drugs. With Jessica only twenty-seven years old, feeling like she was still very young, they did not plan to move to more invasive procedures such as IVF for some time. Facing extremely irregular periods, Jessica took superovulatory drugs during her first cycle at the clinic, but the drugs failed to stimulate any eggs. Switching drugs for a second cycle, Jessica forged ahead, to find that this time she was overstimulated and had too many eggs to safely proceed; the risk of becoming pregnant with multiples was too great. Jessica and Ethan faced a choice that needed an immediate answer: cancel the now high-risk cycle and try again with a lower dosage in an effort to stimulate fewer eggs, or harvest the eggs and convert to an IVF cycle. Forced to confront the IVF question much sooner than they anticipated, they uneasily opted to proceed. Her eggs were extracted and fertilized in the lab. They transferred their sole surviving embryo back to Jessica's womb on day three. A beautiful baby girl was born nine months later.

Paula and Derrick experienced the flip side of the equation. Having suffered a miscarriage and multiple failed attempts at conceptions, they turned to a treatment plan consisting of high levels of superovulatory drugs to be used in combination with IVF. Although the drugs did stimulate the production of eggs, there were not enough to proceed with IVF. Like Jessica and Ethan, they faced an immediate choice. Abandon the cycle altogether as they had the first time, or switch to IUI (intrauterine insemination)—essentially attempting fertilization with a "turkey baster"—which had a risk of multiples. Anxiously, they went ahead with the IUI and Paula became pregnant. Sadly, she miscarried at seven weeks.

In my case, my various doctors and clinics in the United States and the United Kingdom never turned to superovulatory drugs, since I seemed to produce plenty of eggs on Clomid alone—although those eggs did not transform into a viable baby.

In the confrontation between the stream and the rock, the stream
always wins—not through strength, but through persistence.
Anonymous

Go East, Young Lady

The World of Complementary and Alternative Therapies

T he months waiting for my appointment with Dr. Sacks went slowly. While waiting, I turned thirty-three years old. I was still taking Clomid, still not ovulating, and I couldn't help feeling like I was wasting valuable time.

Over tea one day, Melissa, a close friend, former colleague, and fellow type A personality, suggested I look at acupuncture to help induce my period. She'd used it to calm muscle spasms. Another friend, who was a doctor, told me that in Europe, a study had demonstrated an increase in IVF success rates when acupuncture was paired with traditional treatment. And my friend Julie's boyfriend used it for relief of back pain. I had never been one for alternative therapies, but what did I have to lose? At a minimum, perhaps it could help with the dreaded Clomid headaches.

The acupuncture clinic of Dr. Mengda Shu was not at all what I expected, although I am not sure exactly what I thought it would be like. A corporate attorney with a severe needle phobia, I was a bundle of nerves, skepticism, anxiety, and also excitement. Would it help? Would it hurt? Would I faint at the sight of needles? As soon as Dr. Shu greeted me in the welcoming waiting room, a sense of calm blanketed me. It was uncanny. A slim, graceful woman wearing a white lab coat, she exuded confidence and gentleness. Despite the extreme skepticism I brought with me into the room, I trusted her from the minute I met her.

This elegant woman in her fifties moved with a peacefulness that was infectious and intoxicating. She escorted me to a treatment room, deftly extracting my personal and medical history in fluid conversation, without need of the all-too-familiar medical history form. After telling me about her background, her training in China, her experiences in the United States, and a brief but very clear explanation of how acupuncture works, she felt the pulses on both of my wrists.

She proceeded. "Now please stick out your tongue so I may look at it."

My tongue? How bizarre.

I complied. She studied its color, coat, shape, and size, and then rendered a startlingly accurate report of how I was feeling. My tongue apparently also provided a road map for plotting her course down the pincushion that was my body. She poked me full of tiny little (painless!) sterile needles and stood by my side during the treatment, sometimes talking to me, sometimes silent, sometimes gently tweaking my needles. I went into a state of relaxation that is hard to describe, rivaled only by the state of bliss attained after the best massage imaginable. She sent me home with noxious herbal potions that ironically were more painful to drink than the acupuncture needles that I had feared, and told me that I had to be patient.

"Do not expect any results in less than three months," she told me. "But in about three months, we will see progress."

I saw her every Saturday. Amazingly, the headaches went away with each treatment, and stayed away for days. After about a month, Richard mentioned that he couldn't remember the last time I had a headache, or nausea, or any effects from the 150 mg of Clomid I was still taking, and we realized that all my symptoms were gone. Even if the Chinese medicine and acupuncture were not helping me to get pregnant, they were at least the antidote to the dreaded Clomid, enabling me to live a normal life on the pill that Western medicine believed would get me pregnant.

On a Saturday morning in May, three months after I began the weekly appointments that transported me to a land of hopefulness and bliss, and just a week before my coveted appointment with Dr. Sacks, Dr. Shu offered her congratulations. "Your pulses have changed," she beamed.

"What does that mean?" I asked.

"It means you are pregnant."

Silence.

"Pregnant? How?" I had still not had a period. I couldn't be pregnant.

Dr. Shu laughed. "The old-fashioned way," she said. "It is very early, but you are definitely pregnant."

I left her office with my mind in a whirl. She was either brilliant or crazy.

If I was actually pregnant, I was a confirmed believer in acupuncture and traditional Chinese medicine forever. If I was not, should I even continue with the treatments? How could she tell me *that news* and get my expectations up when she couldn't possibly be sure? But she told me she was positive, that the pulses, read by the Chinese for thousands of years as an early indicator of conception, were as certain as a urine test and more accurate in the early days. I wanted to believe her, especially since she had made my headaches go away, but I wasn't convinced. I went straight to a pharmacy, picked up an over-the-counter pregnancy test, and raced home. I drank tons of water, forced myself to take a test.

Negative. I tried to console myself. Richard was away for work for three weeks, and I suddenly missed him desperately. Only he could console me. How could I possibly explain to family and friends the overwhelming disappointment of a negative pregnancy test after having my expectations raised by a Chinese herbal doctor and acupuncturist, who nobody knew I was seeing for a fertility problem that nobody except my parents really knew that I had? I was furious with myself for getting my hopes up.

The rest of the weekend, I waited for my appointment with the storied Dr. Sacks. On Monday, with Richard away, my anxiety and I made our way to the vaunted office. More than fifteen years later, I still remember the waiting room. It was yellow and bright and had a very friendly aura. What I remember most is the women in it—all anxious but hopeful, glancing at one another with tight little smiles and friendly but reserved nods. All there for the same thing. All frustrated. All hoping Dr. Sacks could help us.

I filled out the requisite questionnaire, similar to the many I would later fill out in London, New York, Geneva, Moscow. This was my first, and I remember one important question: "Number of days since last menstrual cycle: _____" Answer: "10+ months." Seeing that number in print drove it home. 10+ months. Something was clearly wrong.

After the obligatory height, weight, and blood pressure checks and changing into the ubiquitous blue paper sheet that masquerades as a robe, I waited for what seemed like an eternity to meet the man himself. Dr. Sacks entered the room with a wonderful smile and a firm handshake. In stark contrast to my first doctor, he was wholeheartedly invested in my admittedly short fertility tale of woe. He made me feel like he had all the time in the world. We would start out with an ultrasound scan, he explained, so that he could take a look at my ovaries and uterus and then we would have a chat about next steps. I lay back on the medical table for my first of what must have totaled nearly one hundred ultrasound scans over the next many years. As Dr. Sacks scanned my ovaries, I tried to make sense of the fuzzy gray scale images in front of me. He then moved over to my uterus, and broke into a smile.

He asked me to raise my head a bit so that he could show me what we were looking at. He pointed at a tiny dark grayish-blackish dot near the inside edge of a paler gray fuzzy oval.

"Do you see that there?" He waited for my hesitant nod. "That is your baby. Congratulations to both of us. That is my fastest success story ever."

Dr. Sacks went on talking for a while. Something about early days, just conceived, too early for a heartbeat, come back in two weeks when the fetus would be more than six weeks . . . I could barely hear him, for the buzz of happiness in my head.

My Chinese acupuncturist was a genius.

It is my belief that many women at the beginning stages of their journey would do well to explore the world of alternative therapies. Western research on acupuncture and infertility is ongoing, and its success rates remain controversial. Yet in light of Chinese research and practice and small Western studies indicating that acupuncture may improve pregnancy rates during IVF and IUI treatment, increase blood flow to the uterus, reduce stress and anxiety levels, improve ovulation among women with PCOS, strengthen the immune system, and decrease chances of miscarriage, it is easy to see why both patients and doctors are increasingly open to it. "[Acupuncture] can allow you to cross the line from infertile to fertile by helping your body function more efficiently, which in turn allows other, more modern reproductive treatments, like IVF, to also work more efficiently," says James Dillard, MD, an acupuncturist, chiropractor, and medical doctor who served as assistant clinical professor at Columbia University College of Physicians and Surgeons, as well as medical director of Columbia's Rosenthal Center for Complementary and Alternative Medicine.[1] And while there are a variety of opinions on its efficacy, there is generally wide agreement that acupuncture is safe and produces no side effects.

Studies show that acupuncture can increase pregnancy rates among patients undergoing fertility treatments,[2] and anecdotally, a great many women credit traditional Chinese medicine (TCM) and acupuncture in varying degrees to their fertility success. Imami, a thirty-eight-year-old petroleum engineer, was apprehensive about acupuncture. It had taken three years and multiple cycles of Clomid to conceive her first child, and when she returned to the fertility clinic for baby number two, after trying to conceive for ten months, her labs were discouraging. Her fertility specialist suggested she try acupuncture and TCM prior to any medicated cycles. To her great surprise, she became pregnant naturally after two months, using acupuncture, herbs, dietary therapy, and supplements. Similarly, thirty-two-year-old Julia was told by her ob-gyn that based on the results of her blood tests (FSH of 47 in addition to her AMH of .03), she had little chance of getting pregnant. She was directed to the same reproductive endocrinologist as Imami and was likewise encouraged to try acupuncture and TCM and then come back to repeat her blood tests before making any further decisions. Like Imami, Julia found herself pregnant after just over two months of acupuncture and TCM and gave birth to a healthy baby. Having returned to it again and again throughout my journey, I for one am a fan.

Western medicine tends to look at treating infertility from the perspective of "something's broken, let's fix it"—generally the fastest and most direct way. Not ovulating? Take Clomid and force the ovulation.

TCM and acupuncture, on the other hand, come from a completely different perspective, in which the body is seen as a complete ecosystem. As in nature, any one element out of balance can throw off the functioning of the system as a whole. The goal of TCM is to work with the body to bring it back into balance, to the point where it operates properly on its own, as opposed to forcing it. In the case of fertility, this entails regulating the hormones and menstrual cycle—rather than manipulating it with drugs—so that conception will occur naturally.[3]

"We fix the ovulatory problems, the egg quality, by fixing the whole system," acupuncturist Jane Gregorie, MS, LAc, FABORM, explains. "If a woman had hypothalamic amenorrhea,* for example, rather than giving her hormones or fertility medications to override her system and force ovulation, the TCM approach would be to nourish a woman's whole body so that her ovaries could function optimally. The TCM approach usually takes longer but works more holistically: by calming the nervous system and providing sustenance for the generation of her own endogenous gonadotropins, ovulation will happen naturally. We nourish the soil before we plant the seed."[4]

This approach reminds me of my recipe analogy, and my own journey. The Western practice of combatting infertility takes all the ingredients that it needs and puts them together. Eggs? Check. Sperm? Check. But the traditional Chinese system focuses on the quality of the ingredients. Are the eggs and sperm of the highest quality they can be, and if not, why not? The emphasis is placed on what can be done to encourage the system to produce better "ingredients," for a successful dish requires not only a good recipe but also high-quality components. Many women trying to get pregnant need both and increasingly look to Eastern and Western methods to aid them.

The Chinese approach to regulating the cycle is comprehensive, seeking to influence the timing of ovulation while at the same time balancing hormones, building and maintaining the endometrial lining, reducing pain and stress, and improving egg quality. Practitioners of TCM employ a variety of tools to achieve these goals, including acupuncture, herbs, supplements, dietary therapy, moxibustion (involving a warmed herbal compound), self-care practices, lifestyle modifications, and techniques like breath work and meditation.[5]

I discovered this myself over the years, seeing practitioners who worked in different countries and had trained in various schools that emphasized diverse elements of the practice and treatment. Following

---

*This means that she was not ovulating because her hypothalamus was not producing enough gonadotropin-releasing hormone.

my initial experience with traditional acupuncture and Chinese herbal teas, Dr. Xiao-Ping Zhai, of the highly regarded Zhai Clinic in London, a pioneer of acupuncture for fertility in the West, introduced me to electroacupuncture, in which a small electric current is passed between acupuncture needles to heighten the effect, and also suggested that I eliminate all cold food from my diet. Louisa Gordon, an eternally optimistic British acupuncturist who treated me throughout numerous IVF cycles, added moxibustion into my mixture; it scared me at first, but I grew to love it. Moxibustion looks like little clumps of mud, but it is actually a nugget of the herb mugwort placed on the body—in my case on my abdomen—and burned close to an acupoint. The heat from the herbal embers is believed to increase the efficiency of the acupuncture.

The practice of TCM is complex, and it is best to find a practitioner well versed not just in TCM and acupuncture but also specifically trained in enhancing fertility. There are active professional associations that maintain lists of member practitioners devoted to teaching, research, and the practice of traditional and holistic Chinese medicine specifically focused on the treatment of reproductive disorders.[6] Unfortunately, I didn't know this when I moved to various places and set out to find myself an acupuncturist. I relied, for better or worse, on old-fashioned trial and error—sometimes, unfortunately, for the worse.

Dr. Randine Lewis, author of the *The Infertility Cure* and *The Way of the Fertile Soul*, summarized the contrast between Eastern and Western perspectives: "Although Western medicine views the reproductive system as an ever-deteriorating disease process waiting for intervention, Chinese medicine employs a different lens. We view the body/mind/spirit as an ever-adaptive system, which, when given appropriate environmental cues, has a miraculous ability to manifest its highest potential."[7]

That adaptive process takes time, a precious commodity for those racing against the biological clock. In an instant-gratification culture in which nearly anything can be ordered on demand twenty-four hours a day, people are not accustomed to being told that a process might take at least six months, as I was told by Dr. Zhai in London after several failures.

In light of this, it was somewhat surprising to find in my experience talk-ing and corresponding with women across America and in Europe that it was the rare exception when a long-term fertility patient did not turn to acupuncture, TCM, or both. When confronted with multiple failures, or an inability to find answers solely within Western reproductive medicine, women are increasingly embracing this ancient Chinese method.

Notably, it is not simply of their own initiative that women are turn-ing to Eastern methods. Cognizant of the increasing body of evidence supporting the efficacy of the treatments, respected fertility clinics are increasingly working with acupuncturists, sometimes bringing them in-house. Perhaps one of the strongest indicators that many Western fertility specialists are acknowledging the efficacy of the Chinese herbal medicines is that they often don't want their patients taking herbs dur-ing an IVF cycle, largely because they do not know how to anticipate and accommodate the effects.

"My favorite patients, and the most dramatic success stories we have," Gregorie tells me, "are those who aren't even candidates for IVF or Western fertility treatments because their FSH is too high or their AMH is too low. I am grateful for the open-minded REs [reproduc-tive endocrinologists] who send these patients to us rather than telling them they have a hopeless case. My favorite physician colleague would say, 'Go see Jane for three months and do whatever she says, and then come back for retesting.' Sometimes these patients conceive naturally in that time frame because they respond to a more subtle, nourishing approach, and I don't doubt that their doc's belief in an intervention that can help them (even if Western medicine cannot) eases their mind, calming their fight-or-flight response so that the reproductive system is bolstered, not paralyzed by fear or hopelessness."[8]

The Science of TCM and Acupuncture

Based on a classical Chinese theory of regulating vital energy flows, or qi, within a body, acupuncture relies on the painless but strategic placement of tiny needles into meridians, or pathways, that span the body from head to toe, nourishing the tissues. Acupuncturists believe the meridians can stagnate, leading to a variety of problems, including infertility. The needles are thought to stimulate certain key energy points that open the pathways and restore a person's physical and emotional balance, enabling the body to function more efficiently.

In the case of fertility, acupuncture is used to regulate a woman's cycle, to encourage egg production, and to improve the chances of a successful IVF cycle by, among other things, increasing blood flow to the ovaries and the uterus.[9] This improved blood flow can help to both nourish the eggs in the ovaries and thicken the lining of the uterus, the intended home of the newly fertilized embryo, increasing the odds of conception. It is also believed to increase sensitivity to gonadotropins, the hormones injected throughout an IVF cycle to stimulate production of eggs.[10]

Acupuncture may also help correct problems with the body's neuroendocrine system, activating the brain to release hormones that will stimulate the ovaries, the hypothalamus and pituitary (known as the HPO axis), and other organs that are involved in reproduction.[11] Additionally, acupuncture has been shown to assist in reducing stress and anxiety, both believed to interfere with getting pregnant, by releasing endorphins in the brain[12]—an effect I happily experienced myself.

In the case of male factor infertility, acupuncture and TCM have been demonstrated in peer-reviewed studies to enhance sperm count, motility (movement), and morphology (shape).[13]

The Western, scientific perspective on why acupuncture might work is—not surprisingly—a bit different. Rather than clearing pathways that have stagnated, some Western practitioners believe the needles stimulate the nerves where they are placed and trigger the release of hormones that may increase a person's pain threshold and increase feelings of euphoria.[14]

"These chemicals either change the experience of pain, or they trigger a cascade of chemicals and hormones which influence the body's own internal regulating system," says Jill Blakeway, acupuncturist and clinic director at the YinOva Center in New York City.[15] With regards to boosting fertility, acupuncture may increase the effectiveness of medications taken to assist ovulation and fertility by working in tandem to increase the level of hormones traveling to the ovaries.[16]

Dr. Raymond Chang, the medical director of Meridian Medical and a classically trained acupuncturist as well as Western-trained medical doctor, and Dr. Zev Rosenwaks, a well-known Cornell University reproductive endocrinologist, found a clear link between acupuncture and brain hormones, demonstrating that acupuncture increases the production of endorphins, which play a role in regulating the menstrual cycle.[17] Interestingly, a team at the University of California, Irvine, examined the effect on the brain while patients received acupuncture treatment on a point on the little toe that was traditionally used by the Chinese to address eye pain.[18] When the point on the foot was stimulated with the needle, the part of the brain that regulates vision lit up. When tested against a "fake" acupuncture point as a control, there was no reaction.

Acupuncture can also improve success rates with IUI. Researchers at Tel Aviv University in Israel found that nearly a third more of the test group conceived when combining IUI with acupuncture and traditional Chinese medicine than the control group, who received no acupuncture or herbal therapy.[19] This may be due in part to effects on sperm; both quality (fewer defects) and quantity of sperm have been shown to increase following acupuncture treatments.[20]

Despite a dearth of large-scale Western studies, several smaller studies and a recent meta-analysis of larger patient groups indicate that both women experiencing infertility due to PCOS and women undergoing IVF are consistently helped by acupuncture treatments, increasing pregnancy rates by more than 50 percent. Men experiencing infertility with no known cause have also been shown to benefit from acupuncture.[21] Additionally, acupuncture performed on the day of an embryo transfer, particularly when women receive acupuncture both before and after the transfer, has been shown to improve IVF success rates.[22] While noting that acupuncture "is not a panacea," Dr. Jamie Grifo, director of the division of reproductive endocrinology at NYU Langone Medical Center and the founder of its fertility center, observed that "it does improve pregnancy rates and quality of life in some people."[23]

Interestingly, while acupuncturists naturally welcome the support of Western studies indicating a positive result from acupuncture treatments on the day of embryo transfer, many in the field believe that longer-term acupuncture in conjunction with whole-systems TCM—typically a personalized acupuncture protocol, together with any combination of moxibustion, Chinese herbal medicine, dietary recommendations, and massage—leads to greater positive overall outcomes than transfer-day acupuncture alone.[24]

The bottom line: the whole-systems TCM led to more births and fewer miscarriages.

You can have the rug pulled out from underneath
you, or learn to dance on a moving carpet.

Anonymous

You Always Remember Your First

The Ups and Downs of Pregnancy and Loss

After what felt like an eternity (which I later learned was more like a nanosecond) of trying to conceive, I finally had exciting news, and no one to share it with, apart from my acupuncturist, as Richard wasn't due home until the end of the week. For days, I sat alone with my exciting secret. I couldn't tell anyone before I told my husband, and I didn't want to tell him over the phone.

Richard finally returned home late Friday evening. I was exhausted, as I was every day then, but I waited up for him, perched on the kitchen stool in our front window, watching for his car from the airport to arrive.

When the black Town Car pulled up, I ran to the door and greeted him with a huge hug. We soon settled down at the kitchen barstools, he with a Scotch in hand, me with an herbal tea.

"I have something to tell you," I said, suppressing a smile.

"I have something to discuss with you too," he replied. "You first."

"I'm pregnant. We're going to have a baby."

Silence. Confusion.

"The Clomid. The acupuncture. The herbal brews. I don't know what it was, but something worked."

"Wow. This is amazing!"

"Due February twelfth," I continued. "Now, what did you want to tell me?"

"They asked me to move to London."

"Whaaaaat? Who? When? Why?"

Richard explained that he had been given an opportunity to go to London, but it was only for six months, maybe a bit more. His firm wanted him to move soon, as early as late June or very early July. As exciting and professionally beneficial as the move would be, however, he felt he'd have to pass it up. He thought it would be too disruptive to our lives and it didn't make sense, especially now given the pregnancy.

To his surprise, I disagreed. "Let's do it," I told him. "Why not? It will be a great adventure. It's a fantastic opportunity for you. We'll love it. We can travel. The baby will be born there. We'll just have to stay a little longer than six months and your firm will have to deal with it. We'll come back after the baby is born."

We discussed the situation late into the night, and over the next days and nights, getting more excited with each iteration. We chatted about it obsessively until the day arrived when it was time for us to go together to see my fertility specialist for a checkup and the all-important six-week scan that hopefully would yield us our first glimpse of our fetus's heartbeat. We still had not told anyone about the pregnancy, and had been counseled to be cautious in our optimism until we saw a heartbeat, at which point the odds of a successful, healthy pregnancy increase dramatically. We waited for our turn in the cheerful, yellow office and then went in for the obligatory vitals, ubiquitous blue robe, and, finally, the scan, with Richard by my side. Unlike the first time I viewed a scan,

I knew exactly what I was looking at when I saw the dark peanut in the pale gray circle-ish shape, throbbing. THROBBING. That was the heartbeat! The doctor showed us that little flashing plus sign on the screen, and the excitement kicked in. We were really having a baby. On (or about) February 12, 2002. That's what the computer said.

We made the final decision to move to London, and, all of a sudden, we had a lot to do. It was early June and we were expected to go by early July. We told our families our double news. We were having a baby (much excitement!) and moving to London for a while (mixed reception).

Following my departure from the California tech firm, I had recently taken a new position at a law firm and had started one week before finding out that I was pregnant and just eleven days before learning that my husband's company wanted him to move to London. Great timing. After only twelve days working at the new firm, I had to go to the head of the corporate department, explain the situation, and ask to be transferred to the London office. It wasn't a complete disaster, but it didn't go as well as I had hoped. He didn't think it was likely in the time frame I was talking about. "Maybe in six months?" he suggested.

Emboldened by the thought of the little throbbing peanut inside me, I told him that wouldn't work for me. Richard and I needed to be on the same continent. I spoke to a few headhunters. These were pre-9/11 days; the economy was booming, and it did not seem like it was going to be too hard to get a job in London. We decided to forge ahead with our plans, with or without my firm's cooperation. Two days later, the head of corporate called to say I could go to London with Richard in July. The stars were finally aligning for us.

The pregnancy seemed to be progressing swimmingly. I was extremely tired but had almost no morning sickness, and Dr. Sacks, seeing no further need for his specialized services, had passed me along to a local ob-gyn practice to monitor my pregnancy until the move. I had my first appointment at the new practice, and the doctor there took blood tests and did another ultrasound scan. All looked great. We saw the heartbeat, still looking strong, and the fetus was growing. This ultrasound machine showed an estimated due date of February 16, 2002. I asked about it, as I expected it to be February 12, 2002. Not to worry, the technician said. Machines can calibrate differently. Everything was fine.

The practice saw me again just before we traveled to England. The doctor wanted to do one more scan before we left, and to review the results of the blood tests. To my surprise, the tests revealed what was described as a small problem. I had an elevated marker for toxoplasmosis.[1] I had no idea what toxoplasmosis was, but my heart started beating rapidly. How could I be learning of a problem the day before the move? The doctor calmly explained that it might be nothing at all, that it was often detected in women with cats in the household (we had three), that it came from kitty litter, and that the markers might be present in my blood from an earlier infection. I was still concerned. The doctor drew more blood to send to a specialized lab in California and promised to call with the results of the blood analysis, which she warned might take weeks. She advised me to find an obstetrician in London right away and to both inform the doctor of the toxoplasmosis risk and get a scan as soon as possible. In parting, she told me not to think at all about the toxoplasmosis. It was probably nothing.

Our good friends Steve and Shelley host an annual Fourth of July pool party that we were determined not to miss. We were planning to go straight from the party to the airport, and so they kindly turned it into a July 4/bon voyage party. We had a spectacular time with family and many of our closest friends, and felt on top of the world. We were finally starting a family, as well as embarking on a new adventure. Although we were not yet at the end of the first trimester, when most people consider it "safe" to reveal the big news, given our multiple scans, heartbeat sightings, and assurances that all looked well, we shared our exciting news with everyone at the party. On the last flight of the night on July 4, we were bound for England. We saw fireworks from the plane as we began our overseas adventure.

Unfortunately, it wasn't exactly the rosy start I had envisioned to our life in London. It was a difficult flight, followed by a bumpy black cab ride to our new home, a super-expensive, super-tiny apartment on Weymouth Street in Marylebone. I arrived nauseous, exhausted, and excessively hormonal. Richard's company had found the apartment and was covering the rent for the six-month stint. Given the exorbitant cost, I had been excitedly expecting a correspondingly lavish apartment. Now don't get me wrong here. I grew up in a lovely, modest, middle-class home in Buffalo, New York, and my parents grew up in the Bronx. During graduate and law school, I had lived in housing so substandard in NYC that my brother, Ken, called the city's office for poison control to complain about the rats. But given the astronomical rent, I'd had visions of those lovely Merchant Ivory period pieces. Instead, we arrived at a tiny, modern, characterless box. I burst into tears. Richard teases me to this day.

I had been told to call the head of my law firm's London office the morning I arrived, but, tired and nauseous, I crawled into bed. I lay there. Until my guilt got the better of me. Before I went to sleep for the rest of the day, I knew I should call the head of the office. His secretary put me on hold. When he came on the line, he said, "Welcome, hope the journey was good, can you come down to the office now?" I couldn't answer. "Do you know the way? Sorry to bring you in today, but I am off on vacation tomorrow so it would be best if you could come in now." Damn. My first morning off a red-eye? The doctors had told me to get lots of rest.

Dejected, I pulled myself out of bed, somehow got myself into a suit, and headed out to the Great Portland Street Tube station, walking slowly in the drizzle past The Portland Hospital for Women and Children, not knowing at the time that it was perhaps the most famous maternity hospital in the United Kingdom, if not the world, and that I would be spending a fair amount of time there in my near future.

After completing the necessary work-related introductions and tasks, I was shown to my new office and promptly began *my* first project—getting myself an ob-gyn and an appointment. Armed with the name of a doctor recommended by my close college friend Kathy, who is an ob-gyn in Boston, I placed my first phone call, hoping for an appointment that week. No, unfortunately, Ms. Maggie,* the doctor I was referred to, was away on a ten-week leave and wasn't taking any new patients. Her receptionist referred me to a colleague, coincidentally also named Ms. Maggie, who couldn't see me until the first week in August, which would be fine because I would be just over twelve weeks, nearing the end of my first trimester. In the meantime, the receptionist would refer me for a scan at an ultrasound clinic.

I went for the scan at the end of that first week in London, eager to get another glimpse of the fetus and make sure everything was OK after the long journey. I was amazed by the ability of reflected sound waves to render an image of the tiny being in my womb. What an immense relief to learn that all was still fine: heartbeat strong and fetus growing. I noticed that the ultrasound machine showed an estimated due date of February 17, 2002. *Strange, another day off*, I thought, but I didn't ask. I thought I would wait until I met my new doctor in early August.

As I settled into work in the heart of the old City of London, I felt healthy and optimistic, and looked forward to meeting my new ob-gyn. My New York Jewish mother called religiously to make sure I was eating enough and getting rest. She'd waited a long time for this grandchild and was as excited as I was.

I never got to meet Ms. Maggie. Less than three weeks later, I was in a meeting at my office and knew something was terribly wrong. I had horrible cramps. Everything was tightening. It hurt so much I had to fight back tears, although in retrospect it is hard to know if the tears were from the pain or from the knowledge that something was seriously wrong. I excused myself and went to the bathroom as calmly as I could, and although I was not entirely surprised, I gasped when I saw the blood

---

*Doctors in the United Kingdom are referred to as Mr., Mrs., or Ms., as the case may be, rather than Dr., unless they have a PhD.

in my underwear. From the bathroom stall I called Richard in a panic. He calmly told me to call the doctor and to try not to worry. I hastily attempted to clean myself up and make my way back to my office without arousing attention. When I called the doctor's office, I was told that she was on vacation but that I could see her partner, Mr. R. I hailed a taxi and went straight to the office.

Upon entering his office on the famed Harley Street, as distraught as I was, I could not help but notice my surroundings. A huge wooden desk with impeccable leather accessories. Oil paintings on the walls. A bronze sculpture. No computer. Sitting in a high-back black leather chair amid an array of nineteenth-century antiques, he greeted me politely, asking how I was, did I like London, wasn't it a dreadful day outside indeed. He reminded me of Peter O'Toole in *The Last Emperor*. I was cramping and terrified of what had just happened, and not in the mood for British pleasantries. After he chatted with me for what seemed like an unbearable amount of time, he sent me off to the Fetal Medicine Centre for an ultrasound scan without even examining me.

I don't remember the walk to the Fetal Medicine Centre, which was just a couple of blocks away, and I don't remember calling my husband to tell him to meet me there, but I must have done both because I somehow got to the center and he showed up some time later. A kind doctor named Dr. Simona took me in for a scan. She didn't need to tell me anything. Novice as I was, the lack of the constant pulse from the ultrasound screen, coupled with the forced, expressionless look on Dr. Simona's face told me all I needed to know. There was no heartbeat. There was no baby. I had known it in my office. I knew it now. But why? What happened? I couldn't bear it. I couldn't accept it. Overwhelmed with grief, I cried and cried. I was actually shocked by how completely grief-stricken I was. I think I took it worse than I had ever taken anything in my life.

Dr. Simona quietly explained that I'd technically had a "missed abortion" as the medical industry cruelly calls it. The fetus, absent a heartbeat, was still inside me; mercilessly true to its name, a "missed abortion" is even missed by the body of one experiencing it, which continues to feel pregnant. It was of little comfort to learn that miscarriages after seeing a heartbeat were rare and that only 1 percent of women suffer "missed abortions."

Later, much later, as the haze started to clear for bits of time and I would wander aimlessly around Regents Park, as I often did, or sit on a park bench staring into space, or sit on my couch as was my habit on the many rainy days, or the days when I simply couldn't get up, I felt guilty. Guilty about all the people I knew who had experienced miscarriages and how little I had understood it. How little attention I had paid. I felt horror at my failure to empathize. I could not possibly have imagined the intensity of the loss a person could feel for a life that had not yet been born.

It took me a few days to want to talk to anyone. At the office, I told only the office manager, Jackie, who was incredibly sympathetic, and my two new friends and colleagues, Susan and Kathryn, with whom I spent virtually all of my time at work. Susan was pregnant at the time, and it was particularly painful to tell her, especially as it was early in her pregnancy as well.

I called my parents and could barely talk to them through my tears. Everyone was shocked. Everyone, that is, except my close friend Kathy, the ob-gyn. I could tell that she wasn't surprised. When I pressed her, she hesitated and then confessed that she had been worried about me.

"Why?" I asked, confused.

"Because your due date kept slipping. Your due date should never slip by five days. The fetus wasn't growing properly. They should have told you."

I was stunned. There were warning signs. She explained that at that stage of early development, a difference of five days was very significant, and that she had suspected that there was a problem with the embryo, very likely a chromosomal problem.

The next part of our conversation, on the other hand, did surprise her. Kathy explained to me that the doctor would most likely be planning to test the chromosomes when he did the dilation and curet-tage, known as a D&C, but that I should ask about it and make sure that they were definitely planning to do so, so that we could learn from this loss. I told her that Mr. R had strongly counseled against a D&C when he had called a few hours after the scan, and wanted me to wait for the dead fetus to pass naturally, a process that sounded scary, painful, and messy. In addition to the physical horror, I did not welcome the emo-tional toll of walking around knowing that I was carrying a dead baby. It had been panicking me.

"Whaaaaat?" Kathy exclaimed. "That's crazy." She thought I should get the D&C right away. Not only did she think it was emotionally bet-ter for me, but we were likely to get useful information about the fetus, and it would have physical benefits as well. I would know that I had been emptied of all the retained products and I would begin to heal and my cycle restart. She emphasized that I was at risk of infection from the dead tissue inside me, and that I had no idea if or when it would come out. We also knew from the ultrasound that the miscarriage, di-agnosed at eleven weeks, six days into the pregnancy, likely occurred at approximately nine weeks. Her feeling was that if it had not spontane-ously evacuated by now, it was not going to. I called the doctor several times. I practically begged him to do a D&C. He insisted that I wait two weeks. I grew to hate the sound of his voice, his repeated denials of my request for the procedure.

Richard urged me to call another doctor. Kathy urged me to call another doctor. My mother urged me to call another doctor. She had never trusted a doctor that didn't have a computer. I couldn't act. I couldn't explain it, but I felt paralyzed.

Finally, the day came that Mr. R had scheduled the D&C at The Portland. I was relieved, almost strangely excited, to be getting this dead alien being out of my body after two horrendous weeks of waiting. I was not, however, looking forward to seeing Mr. R again. It turns out I needn't have worried about it. He never showed up. He had a family emergency, and Richard and I waited anxiously for news of what would happen next.

Eventually, a dashing, charming gentleman in a tuxedo popped in to introduce himself. He would be filling in for Mr. R. We must excuse him, he had been on his way to a gala of some sort, when he got diverted to perform my procedure. He would just scrub up and be with us in a jiffy. We were both relieved—he was wonderful. The procedure went smoothly, and when I woke my newest doctor, who happened to be the Surgeon-Gynaecologist to Queen Elizabeth II's Royal Household, was there, regaling us with his stories. I loved him and wanted him to be my doctor. He politely declined. He couldn't think of taking a patient from Mr. R. As suddenly as he arrived, he was off, and we were left alone with our reality—sitting in a recovery room in a posh maternity hospital surrounded by mothers and babies when we had just lost ours. It was time to get out of there and refocus on the future.

Several weeks later, I received a fax at my office from Washington, DC. Not to worry about the toxoplasmosis, it said. It was a marker from an old infection and was not a threat to the pregnancy. I didn't have long to dwell on it. It was September 11, 2001.

Another two weeks later, I received the following letter from Mr. R:

> I have now received the Chromosomes results on the products of conception and these show that the fetus was abnormal. The chromosome showed an extra X chromosome which would be the cause of the miscarriage. This should not be repeated in a future pregnancy and is a one-off.
>
> I look forward to seeing you soon.

That was our last communication.

The cause of my first miscarriage at the age of thirty-three was a chromosomal abnormality in the fetus, believed to be the culprit in as many as two-thirds to three-quarters of first trimester miscarriages.[2] The most common cause of miscarriage, a chromosomal abnormality in the embryo is generally thought to be a random event resulting from errors in cell division in the egg, sperm, or just forming embryo. This kind of miscarriage is termed "sporadic" (as opposed to "recurrent"), and is experienced by a quarter of all women, the vast majority of whom will go on to bear healthy children.

In my case, it likely wasn't random at all but due to a whole host of factors that we had yet to discover. Neither was it to be a "one-off" event, as my doctor had assumed.

A journey of a thousand miles begins with a single step.

Lao Tzu

5

Baby Steps

Minimally Invasive Treatment

It was a new world order now. As my country back home marched its way to an invasion of Afghanistan in the fall of 2001, I set my mind on those things within some semblance of my control. The task now was not just getting pregnant—it was staying pregnant. And I couldn't get pregnant soon enough. The doctors told me to wait three months before trying again. It seemed like forever. Friends I had grown up with, studied with, and worked with were getting pregnant, and it didn't help my mental state that I suddenly seemed to be getting invited to baby showers or first birthday parties on a regular basis. My pregnant colleague, Susan, who was now a close friend, grew bigger and more beautiful each week. Her due date was a week before what had been my own. I was genuinely happy for her and her husband. But I feared I would not be able to get through the birth of their baby without unbearable sadness.

When allowed to restart my efforts, I approached the task of getting pregnant with the zeal of the type A lawyer that I was. Encouraged by Susan, I was now in the care of her doctor, the affable and ever-so-handsome Mr. Jeffrey Braithwaite, also on the famed Harley Street in London. A bit of a cross between Hugh Grant and Colin Firth, he made visits to his office as comforting as reading a Jane Austen novel. As I sat in the Wedgwood blue chair in the elegant wood-paneled reception room, I smiled to myself thinking how pleased my mother would be; she had, after all, named me after Elizabeth Bennett.

Not yet as convinced as I that there was something very wrong, at the start, Mr. Braithwaite was confident we would succeed together. The course of action he proposed was similar to the original course set by my first gynecologist in DC; the only difference was in timing. Because my period had never returned after my first miscarriage, Mr. Braithwaite decided to induce a cycle with norethisterone (a synthetic progestogen) and then begin Clomid, but his plan was for me to start the Clomid on day two of my cycle, continuing until day six, in contrast with the previous schedule of days five through nine of each cycle. Mr. Braithwaite felt that merely switching to days two through six of my cycle would produce a better result, which it did. Fortunately for me, he believed 150 mg was a bit excessive, and suggested we start at 100 mg to reduce my unbearable headaches.

It was November again, Thanksgiving upon us, when I restarted the Clomid. I couldn't shake the feeling that I had lost a whole year in the blink of an eye. Dreading the side effects, I was determined that this time I would at least learn more about my cycle. Susan had given me a book, *Taking Charge of Your Fertility*, which became my bible. It explained so many mysteries of the human female body. How had I made it through high school and college and graduate school and law school and not learned any of this? The book was fascinating. One of its prime directives was for every woman to learn her own cycle through charting.

Charting required me to take my basal body temperature every morning as soon as I woke up and to pay careful attention to my body and its relationship to what was going on in my life. Every day, I meticulously wrote down the time that I woke up, my body temperature, the state of my cervical fluid, and anything else that was going on that might be relevant—travel, exercise, illness, stress, alcohol, anything that might affect my cycle. Essentially Bridget Jones's diary if Bridget were trying to get pregnant. The theory was that this charting would help illuminate the timing of my ovulation (essential information in the quest to get pregnant) and would also help to detect a pregnancy at the earliest possible moment through identifying changes in body temperature. Charting became an obsession for me, and an annoyance for Richard. For charting brought with it the demise of carefree, spontaneous sex.

I was still using my Baby Computer, and the fact that the two sets of information coincided very nicely every month reinforced my belief and confidence in both. Mr. Braithwaite, on the other hand, didn't place much faith in either. He placed far more stock in the ultrasound machine in his office that he used to scan my ovaries to look for growing follicles, starting about a week into my cycle and continuing every other day or every third day until ovulation. The triple-feedback loop further built my confidence in the Computer, which was infallible in indicating my ovulation, as well as my belief that I would soon be pregnant.

One thing that most doctors fail to warn patients about is the toll that all these baby-making attempts will take on their romantic lives. When going to all the trouble, not to mention the expense, of taking Clomid or other superovulatory drugs, a couple cannot afford to be cavalier with their sex life. Intercourse must be carefully timed and sometimes rationed. Sex now has a purpose, and no shot at having a baby should be squandered. It took a long time for Richard to adjust to our new reality of sex as dictated by my ob-gyn. "I need you home Tuesday and Thursday this week, period," are not the romantic words most husbands dream of hearing.

Miraculously, thankfully, joyfully, it all worked on the third cycle.

On February 5, 2002, I happily discovered I was pregnant again. Just six days later, one day before my ill-fated first due date, Susan and her husband, Rob, welcomed their beautiful baby Isabelle at The Portland. I went to see them and their new baby that afternoon. Isabelle was absolutely breathtaking. Susan looked exhausted but radiant, her smile peaking through her shiny black hair as she bent down to hand Isabelle to Rob. Clichéd as it may sound, Rob was beaming, his eyes sparkling as he gently lifted her tiny fingers, one by one. I was relieved to find that I was genuinely happy for them. And they were as thrilled—and I suspect, thankful—as I was that I was pregnant again.

Five weeks later, filled with a strange blend of excitement and dread, Richard and I went for our first ultrasound to see the baby and hear the little pulsing heartbeat, which can usually be picked up at around five or six weeks after conception. As Mr. Braithwaite began the scan, the gray fuzz starting to take shape, his expression became as still as the screen. Although Richard had no idea, I knew right away. There was no heartbeat.

It was my second miscarriage—or missed abortion—in less than six months.

After waiting the requisite three months, Mr. Braithwaite was ready to plunge back in. Clomid, cycle charting, ultrasound scans, Baby Computer, acupuncture. We did everything "right," but this time there was no pregnancy.

By New Year's, even the eternally optimistic Mr. Braithwaite agreed that it was time to move on to intrauterine insemination (IUI). After three harrowing Clomid plus IUI cycles (including an exhausting and stressful 5:00 a.m. trip to Heathrow Airport with my husband so he could produce a "sample" in the restroom at the optimal moment, followed by my frantic rush back to my fertility clinic by train and taxi to get the precious vial there in time), like the vast majority of others trying to conceive with IUI, I was not pregnant.

Intrauterine Insemination

If sex on a schedule seems a romantic buzzkill, it feels downright uto-pian when instead a father-to-be is reduced to producing his contribu-tion in a cup in a private room filled with girlie magazines, while his female partner lies on a table with her feet in stirrups. Welcome to the world of intrauterine insemination, or IUI, also known colloquially as artificial insemination, the first step into the world of assisted reproduc-tive technology.

When Clomid and superovulatory drugs alone fail to produce a baby, the vast majority of fertility specialists turn to IUI, largely because it is the least invasive and usually the least expensive form of assisted reproductive technology (ART).[1]

The relatively low cost reflects the fact that IUI is a fairly simple procedure. IUI is almost always used in conjunction with ovulation stimulation (Clomid or superovulatory drugs) and close monitoring. The insemination will be scheduled twenty-four to thirty-six hours after the LH surge that indicates ovulation is about to occur (either naturally or more often, following a trigger shot). On the day of in-semination, the hopeful dad (i.e., sperm provider) will preferably go to the lab or clinic to produce a fresh semen sample, which will then be washed and processed, separating the strongest and fastest swimmers from the rest. It doesn't always go according to plan though. I've spoken with women whose partners have obtained their samples in restaurants, offices, and Starbucks restrooms, wherever he needed to be during the fifteen- to thirty-minute window the doctor specified. When timing is everything, there are few hurdles one won't jump through to get the goods to the lab on time. After the sample is prepared, the star sperm are inserted into the womb through a catheter, in a relatively quick and painless procedure.

While IUI is financially the only option available to many, unfor-tunately, it is also among the least successful of the procedures, with a success rate according to some studies of as low as 10 percent per cycle, even among women under thirty-five. According to Resolve: The National Infertility Organization, many studies have shown that the use of IUI in women older than forty, even when paired with Clomid, does not improve pregnancy rates over not doing anything at all. Similarly, in the case of women who do not ovulate regularly, compared to intercourse, IUI does not improve the chance of pregnancy. Recognizing its failure to significantly improve pregnancy rates, the British National Institute for Health and Care Excellence (NICE) no longer recommends IUI for women with unexplained infertility or for male infertility problems, unlike in the United States, where IUI is still seen as appropriate treatment. To the contrary, IUI is only recommended in the United Kingdom in very specific cases such as sperm donation, where a physical problem prevents intercourse, or when a parent is attempting to prevent passing on a communicable disease.

I spoke with dozens of women who were experiencing fertility problems and turned to IUI. Only one had a baby to show for it.

Once you put human life in human hands, you have
started on a slippery slope that knows no boundaries.

Leon Kass

The Big Guns

Moving on to IVF

*A*pprehensive, although also a bit excited, I went off to see Mr. P, the fertility specialist recommended by Mr. Braithwaite. Although just down the road, Mr. P's office lacked the warmth I had grown accustomed to. The image Mr. P projected—with his carefully balanced combination of Hermès tie, Montblanc pen, office full of Louis IV furniture, and of course, the Porsche 911 out front—reinforced my misconception that financial success must correlate with fertility success. After a very brief conversation, Mr. P told me that he thought IVF was "the only route for me." He suggested, however, that prior to beginning my first cycle, I go for testing at the world renowned Recurrent Miscarriage Clinic at St. Mary's Hospital for further investigation and to rule out potential complications. Of course, as with all things fertility related, despite

being armed with a reference letter implying a sense of urgency, I had
to wait months for my appointment.

I had never heard of antiphospholipid syndrome before the day I
was diagnosed with it by Mr. Raj Rai during our first visit to the Recurrent Miscarriage Clinic. This time, I had insisted that Richard cancel a
business trip so that he could come with me. The wait had made me so
tense I was afraid I wouldn't be able to think straight or retain the salient
information. It hadn't occurred to me that I wouldn't even understand
the words. I repeated after Mr. Rai, "antiphospholipid syndrome," which
he proceeded to tell me was a fancy word for blood clots. I had a condition in which my blood clotted too much, and this was associated with
higher rates of miscarriage. Brilliant, as they say in England. We had an
answer, again. As with the charming doctor who performed my first
D&C, I begged him to be my doctor. But no, he could only pass along
treatment recommendations and assure me that he was optimistic that
our next pregnancy would be successful without further need of him.
He warmly shook our hands as he offered to summarize his diagnosis
and recommended course of action in a letter to Mr. P, and then bade
us farewell.

"Fantastically good news!" Mr. P told me at my next appointment,
as he read the letter out loud:

" 'She appears to have a thrombotic aetiology to her miscarriages.
She has an elevated level of Factor VIII: an impaired response to activated
protein-C and thrombo-elastography demonstrates her to have a raised
pre-pregnancy clot strength and an impaired fibrinolytic response.'

"You have antiphospholipid syndrome," he told me as he put the letter down. "Blood clots."

"Is that all?" I asked timidly. "It sounded like a bit more than that."

"No, just medical jargon for blood clots," Mr. P replied.

I asked him to break it down for me. I wanted to understand the diagnosis. The "thrombotic aetiology" to my miscarriages meant that I had
blood clots. The "impaired fibronolyitc response" referred to an impair-
ment in the system that is meant to prevent blood clots from growing

and becoming problematic. The blood clots were actually symptoms of the antiphospholipid syndrome (APS), which he explained was an auto-immune disorder that occurs when a person's immune system produces abnormal antibodies that mistakenly attack fats called phospholipids in the blood. This process makes the person's blood stickier and more likely to clot in arteries and veins.

"The good news?" I asked, a bit baffled.

Now that we had an answer, we had a way forward, I was told. A simple blood thinner, in the form of heparin shots daily, would prevent any further miscarriage.

Upon hearing the news, Mr. P urged us to go straight to IVF.

The world of assisted fertility is rife with analogies, with one of the most common being that of the slippery slope. The arguments tend to sound like this: If you allow gender selection, people will start asking for blond-haired blue-eyed babies.[1] If you allow surrogacy, women will opt for a surrogate to avoid getting fat.[2] If you allow a procedure that enables a woman with mitochondrial disease to have a healthy baby, it opens the door to radical genetic engineering.[3]

Of course, these are valid ethical concerns and must be thought about very carefully in crafting regulations for our society that provide healthy, safe, and ethical guidelines. But from a real-world perspective, most slippery-slope analogies fail to convince me. My interviews with numerous women and couples reinforced my belief that few, if any, would opt for IVF if they didn't have to, would choose not to carry their own baby to escape putting on weight, or would go through an invasive procedure that involves using DNA from a third party simply to create a designer baby.

Giving voice to frustration no doubt felt by celebrities—and noncelebrities—who faced similar criticism of very personal decisions about having a baby, model Chrissy Teigen, when confronted with hostile comments about her choice, together with husband, John Legend, to select a baby girl when undergoing IVF after years of fertility problems, tweeted: "I also picked the embryo with a taste for bacon, a knack for magic and size 7 feet so she can always find shoes."[4]

People turn to these technologies because they *need* them to have a healthy baby.

From my perspective as a patient, the journey through assisted fertility is more akin to a winding jungle path with hidden pitfalls, presenting moments when one has to decide to cross a rickety bridge, or even worse, to swing across by a rope with a hope and a prayer, or else admit defeat and turn back. Of course, there are lots of slippery slopes along that path, and sometimes, in sliding down toward the next bridge, you don't even notice that your resolve, your goals, your tolerance, your strength may have changed while navigating your journey.

Virtually every woman with whom I spoke had a resistance point, a hesitation to crossing that next bridge. For many it was IVF itself. For others it was immunotherapy, or genetic testing, or using an egg donor.

Paula and Derrick hit the first major bump in their road when confronted with the recommendation of an egg donor. Initially favoring adoption, this was a difficult mental leap for Derrick, particularly given his, as well as Paula's, Catholic upbringing and family pressures. They had a further challenge when confronted with a need for a surrogate, and had to work their way through emotional issues in addition to pragmatic ones, such as financing such a complicated and expensive endeavor. Jessica and Ethan's resistance stemmed not from the radical fertility treatments but rather from the constant invasive testing and retesting required by her clinic, much of which they viewed as time wasting and unnecessary. Sarah and Evan, a couple in their early thirties who live in Boston, hesitated before opting for IVF, initially not comfortable with that type of intervention; they hit their next obstacle when contemplating intravenous immunoglobulin transfusions, a controversial therapy.

My first challenging decision point was agreeing to try IVF. My hesitation wasn't religious or ethical, as it is for many. It was practical.

While I had difficulty getting pregnant, I had done so twice, and I just couldn't see how IVF was the answer for me. Mr. P, of course, didn't agree with my amateur analysis and, presumably based on Mr. Rai's anti-phospholipid diagnosis, pushed us to go straight to IVF. But I wasn't totally convinced. I couldn't see how IVF held the answer for me.

Instead of immediately jumping at his suggestion, as had been our previous pattern with every doctor, Richard and I decided to hold off on IVF. We were about to head to a tiny village in the South of France, for a vacation with some friends. I wanted to be away from everything involved in the fertility business—the Clomid, the charting, the invasive tests, the near-daily ultrasounds.

Well, almost everything. I couldn't part with one device—the fertility monitor.

The way some people are addicted to their smartphones, I was addicted to my Baby Computer, which I viewed as a talisman. Cori, the friend who had given it to me, had conceived and given birth to healthy babies, as had the friend who had given it to her (and, as would the women to whom I would eventually pass it on).

We had a wonderful wine-laden French vacation with our friends (and lots of unpasteurized cheese) as I peed on a stick and inserted it in the computer religiously every morning, checking to see if my fertility level was low, high, or peak. I returned tanned, relaxed, and healthy, and just a few weeks later, found out I was pregnant, without needing IVF. I started the blood-thinning shots that day. Knowing that the heparin shots were going to solve my miscarriage problems, I was pregnant, confident, and truly glowing. I had a wonderful month of September.

My exuberance was short-lived. One month later, I started bleeding. I called the Recurrent Miscarriage Clinic and literally begged for an appointment with anybody on the staff, explaining that I feared I was about to have my third miscarriage. My desperation failed to convince the woman on the other end of the phone, who informed me that I would have to have had three complete miscarriages before I qualified for their care, as they only treated *recurrent* miscarriage patients.

By the end of the week, I'd had "a complete miscarriage." I qualified for the clinic's care now that I no longer needed it. It was devastating. I had been so sure that we had discovered the cause of the miscarriages as well as the solution. Numb from the emotional pain, I don't remember much else about it.

But the third miscarriage was all the convincing I needed. Although I didn't fully accept the logic of why my odds of keeping a baby conceived through IVF were greater than those of a baby conceived naturally, I nevertheless bowed to the pressures from Mr. P to try it. I was tired of doing this on my own, and I didn't think I could take another miscarriage, either emotionally or physically. It was a lot of work managing my own health care and keeping it together at the office, the year before I was to be up for partner at a major international law firm. And I was increasingly depressed. Just getting out of bed was difficult. Two years of working so hard to become and stay pregnant was taking its toll.

Deciding to go down the path of IVF felt like a burden was being lifted.[5] I was surrendering my body and medical care to the pros, and if they got me pregnant, surely they were responsible for keeping me pregnant? (It turns out not: for most fertility clinics, conception is the end of the line.)

In early January 2004, with Christmas decorations still glittering along the streets of London, we embarked on our first IVF cycle.

IVF Basics

The goal of IVF, as practiced in the United States and the United Kingdom over the last thirty-five years, is to hormonally stimulate production of as many eggs as possible, extract the eggs from a woman's ovaries, fertilize them in a lab, and place one or more fertilized embryos back into the woman's uterus. I call this, quite unoriginally, the "needle in the haystack" approach, as it was described this way to me by a half dozen or so doctors. They are looking for the one (or two or three) good egg(s) from a pile they have procured through ovarian stimulation. While technology developed over the last two decades can now shed light on the quality of the embryos, it used to be that embryos were judged by appearance alone—size, shape, the extent of fragmentation. In many clinics, this is still how embryos are selected: by appearance under a microscope and how many days they survive.[6]

My IVF initiation began in a small white examination room in Mr. P's Victorian mansion on Harley Street. Eunice, the compassionate nurse in charge of my care, flitted about the room speaking quickly but very clearly and precisely in her comforting British accent. I wondered why she was whirling about, until she turned to face me with a handful of syringes and a few little glass bottles that would have been ador- able if they weren't so threatening sitting on their clinical metal tray. "Right. . . . Now"—she looked me straight in the eye—"let's teach you how to do your injections properly."

She explained each step to me. Some injections came in easy- to-dispense preloaded pens, while others were much more "self-serve." As is common in conventional IVF, I was to begin, counterintuitively, with birth control pills. I can think of few things more frustrating than to be forced to take the Pill after literally years of trying to get preg- nant, but, as I have been told time and again, that's the protocol. The goal is to essentially stop the menstrual cycle to restart and control it. Five days after stopping the pills, I was to start poking myself with fol- licle stimulating hormone (FSH), necessary to stimulate the follicles in my ovaries to develop into the beautiful eggs we were all hoping for. Thankfully, the Puregon I was prescribed, a brand of recombinant FSH (also known as Gonal-f or Follistim, among others), came in a very easy-to-use dispenser called the Puregon Pen.[7] I have long been a fan of good packaging and stylish little kits—yes, I take the fancy shampoo and lotions from nice hotels—and the Puregon Pen didn't disappoint. The bright yellow-and-blue pen, hardly intimidating, was housed in an appropriately serious blue box, which conveniently held the cartridges and instructions too. Eunice taught me how to twist the dial to dispense

150 IUs, my daily dosage, and how to change the cartridge when the first was empty. Then came the main event. In her no-nonsense way, she showed me how to pinch the fat around my abdomen, hold the pen at exactly the right angle, and slowly inject myself. Not as bad as I had feared. Thinking I was done, I started to get up from my chair.

"Good, that's the first step done then," she said. "Did you need some water?" she asked as she saw me rise.

"Uh, no, just the ladies'," I replied, embarrassed that I thought it was that simple.

When I returned, we moved on to Orgalutran, a brand name for ganirelix, which is a gonadotropin-releasing hormone (GnRH) antagonist, meaning that it blocks the function of GnRH, which starts the process of ovulation. Its very important function was to prevent premature ovulation of these wonderful eggs we were cooking in my ovaries. The Orgalutran is also a subcutaneous injection, meaning that it goes under the skin and is relatively easy to inject as precision is not essential. Eunice suggested that we place this one in my thigh. She advised me that the doctor would tell me when to start that one, probably five or six days after starting the Puregon.

Then came the big gun. "The trigger shot," she said gravely. "It is critical that you get this right." No pressure there. The Profasi,[8] or human chorionic gonadotropin (HCG), injection controls the final maturation and ovulation of the eggs. Injected thirty-six hours before the intended egg collection, the timing of this shot is critical, Eunice intoned again. "If it's too soon, you may ovulate prematurely and all of your eggs will be lost. Too late and the eggs may be difficult to collect and you could have fewer available." And that wasn't all. I had to mix this injection at home from a powder—with no mistakes of course—and the concoction was then to be injected by my husband through a very large needle into a muscle in precisely the right spot in my buttocks. But not to worry, Eunice assured me kindly. When the time came, she would mark the spot for my husband with an X by Sharpie.

Miraculously, ours was a perfect cycle, we were told, and it wasn't even too unpleasant, once I got used to giving myself the dreaded shots, with needles significantly less friendly than the acupuncture needles to which I'd grown accustomed. I had twenty follicles, which produced sixteen eggs, that in turn led to twelve fertilized embryos, of which seven were high quality—fabulous numbers, they said. After enduring just over two weeks of blood tests, hormone injections, ultrasounds, and the final, daunting intramuscular injection delivered by Richard into my derriere, two grade I, two-day-old embryos were transferred to my uterus. Unlike in the treatment of most other women, my shots didn't stop then. On the day of the embryo transfer, I began my daily shots of Clexane (the blood thinner for my antiphospholipid syndrome) into my tummy. Everyone was optimistic.

I thought the hard part was over, but unfortunately, we were only halfway to the finish line. No one warns you that the "two-week wait" is the most excruciating part of IVF. Through the weeks of shots, I was too busy and focused keeping track of my daily calendar and too stressed about getting everything right to think much about the outcome. Also, I think that taking such active steps as shooting yourself with a needle every day is oddly empowering; "taking control" of my reproductive system made me feel optimistic that it would work. Then, abruptly, all the activity comes to a stop and the only job is to wait, leaving enormous amounts of time for anxiety to build.

I don't know if any woman undergoing IVF actually makes it to the clinic blood test without testing at home first, but I certainly didn't. Nor did Paula or Jessica or Sarah or any of the women I spoke with. Nina, a physician from Boston, was so anxious she sometimes tested multiple times per day. I bought so many home pregnancy tests, Richard and I joked that we should have bought stock in the company.

Finally, the day arrived. It worked! I became pregnant for the fourth time. I so wished we had done this sooner. It wasn't so bad. Why had I been resistant to IVF?

Less than a month later, the day before my first ultrasound scan was scheduled, I began to spot. Panicked, I called Eunice. She assured me that spotting was normal, especially with IVF, and that I should come in for a scan. But I knew. I was pregnant no longer. My fourth miscarriage in less than three years. Devastation, frustration, anger, tears. We had done everything right. What was the problem?

Fortunately, the clinic had frozen five good-looking embryos, which my doctor suggested we use in the next cycle. But, of course, we had to wait. The one constant in fertility treatment, the inevitable mandate we could never escape, was the wait—this time, a few months before we could attempt our frozen embryo transfer. At least the embryo transfer was supposed to be much easier on my body.

Frozen Embryo Transfer

Since the early 1980s, when IVF was in its relative infancy, excess embryos produced during a cycle have for the most part been frozen, through a slow freezing process, for future use. Although many healthy children have been born of slow-frozen embryos, as many as 40 percent of embryos were lost during the thawing process, and those that survived experienced substantially lower implantation rates than those of fresh embryos.

A new method of ultrafast freezing, called vitrification, has radically improved post-thaw survival rates and pregnancy rates. First introduced in Spain in 2007, and in use in an increasing number of US clinics since 2008, vitrification has boosted survival rates of frozen embryos from 60 percent to as much as 95 percent.[9] Pregnancy success rates with blastocyst vitrification are so high, rivaling those of fresh blastocysts, that doctors are now increasingly turning toward "freeze all" cycles, particularly when used in conjunction with preimplantation genetic testing.

With a frozen embryo transfer, whatever the freezing method, there is no need to stimulate egg production as with traditional IVF. Rather, the challenge when working with a frozen embryo is to trick the body into preparing to welcome the embryo as it would in a normal ovulatory cycle, without ovulation actually occurring. As with a fresh cycle, this is done with hormones. Eunice instructed me again, and thankfully this time it was a lot easier than the first, as there were barely any injections. I began once more with birth control pills, cringing each morning as I swallowed my pill before brushing my teeth. The day before I stopped the Pill, I began sniffing Synarel (also known as nafarelin) twice a day to downregulate my cycle. A GnRH agonist, Synarel stops the production of natural hormones that control the release of eggs from the ovaries, and is best ingested through nasal passages. Although it wasn't my favorite smell, I was very grateful that it was not a shot. After about three weeks of sniffing Synarel every morning and night, I cut down to once a day, and added in a daily tablet of Progynova, a form of oral estrogen critical to the most important step of a successful transfer—thickening the uterine lining, known as the endometrium, to receive the embryo.

In the first step toward pregnancy, the tiny embryos implant in the uterine wall; if the lining of the uterine wall is too thin, the embryos don't tend to stick around. As I began preparing my body for the frozen embryos, I took Progynova exactly as prescribed, but my body didn't respond; my uterine lining remained too thin to attempt to implant the embryos. We abandoned the cycle. I was crushed. How could we possibly have a new problem now? We waited (again). We tried (again). The lining was too thin (again). We abandoned (again). I was at wit's end. At this point, worried about my physical as well as my emotional health, Richard, who had long been a fan of adoption, was ready to move on. But I wasn't there yet.

And then, just when it couldn't possibly get any worse, it did. In the middle of what had been a delicious, celebratory dim sum lunch with clients, my phone rang. It was Mr. P. I excused myself, hoping he might have good news—a new treatment? A new idea? No, he was calling to apologize. "I'm sorry," he said, in his posh voice. "There's been a mix-up. The lab didn't get my message that the cycle was canceled, and well, it seems they have gone and thawed all your embryos by mistake. But the good news is your next cycle of IVF is on me."

Destroyed. My five high-quality embryos, our potential little babies:

gone. I don't know which was stronger, my fury or my despair. I had to return to a plate full of dumplings and somehow put on a smile for my clients. Richard and I easily could have sued, as we were urged to time and again by people who understood the magnitude of the loss. But we didn't want to. We just wanted our baby. We agreed to do the free IVF cycle with Mr. P as soon as medically permissible.

There's something you must remember . . . you're braver than you believe, and stronger than you seem, and smarter than you think.

Christopher Robin to Winnie-the-Pooh

Understanding Modern ART
Key Aspects of Assisted Reproductive Technology

*E*very woman struggling to have a baby has that "aha" moment when she takes charge of her fertility. For some, it is after one failure. For others, it follows years of fruitless trying. For me, it happened four miscarriages and three years into my journey.

I was lying alone in a hospital bed in Central London, cradling my swollen abdomen, which hours earlier had *forty* eggs removed in my second attempt at IVF. I was nervous. More nervous than I wanted to admit to my husband, or even to myself, I suppose. Staring at the ceiling, I wondered how I had gone so quickly from the heights of optimism about what Mr. P had called an "amazing" IVF cycle to the intense anxiety and discomfort I was experiencing because of my ovarian hyperstimulation (OHSS). After the blow of the thawed embryos, we had been so hopeful that this next (free) IVF cycle would work. Far less intimidating the second time around, we repeated essentially the same protocol as before, but with higher dosages of fertility drugs.[1] My estrogen levels had soared, and Mr. P instructed me to "coast" for a few days, refraining from ingesting or injecting any hormones, while my estrogen level came down to an acceptable range. We then continued as planned. We had *forty* follicles, which produced twenty-six eggs, nineteen of which fertilized. Two were transferred to my womb, and ten were frozen.

I had read about OHSS, and signed the requisite waiver acknowledging the risks. It sounded dreadful—with complications ranging from an excessively swollen uterus to possible death—but it also seemed like something that happened to someone else. Not to me. In fact, the whole thing felt like it was surreal. How was this happening? This was not the trajectory of the life I envisioned when I had joyously married Richard nearly five years earlier.

After returning home from my thoroughly exhausting and depressing hospital stay, I *finally* decided to take the situation into my own hands. My first act was to start to do my own serious research into IVF. And I was shocked by what I learned. Mr. P's techniques were out of date. He was transferring embryos on their second day of development rather than on day three or day five, when the embryos were much more mature and had demonstrably higher rates of success. And he was judging embryos on appearance alone, an antiquated practice now that state-of-the-art testing had become available. When I asked him pointed questions about his protocol versus newer advancements, he couldn't respond. It was time to wake up and take charge of my fertility.

My friend Kathy, the ob-gyn, had heard enough too. One of the smartest and most caring people I know, it was maddening for her to have a close friend with a problem broadly in her field receiving care that she felt was substandard. And to make matters worse, she was an ocean away, hearing my unsophisticated medical reports secondhand and unable to direct my care. Between my first ob-gyn's reluctance to perform a D&C, four miscarriages in a row, and now my fertility specialist causing ovarian hyperstimulation syndrome, she insisted that it was time to come visit her in Boston. Although Kathy is not specialized in fertility (she is a high-risk neonatal expert), she had friends who were, and was confident that I would receive better care at her hospital, Brigham and Women's Hospital.

I flew to Boston a bundle of nerves and excitement. I was hopeful that Kathy's friend, Dr. Rachel Ashby, would have answers for me, but fearful that if she didn't, it might be the end of my road. And I knew I wasn't ready to quit yet. Meeting Rachel was a game changer, although not in the way I had necessarily hoped. She didn't hold the golden key. She didn't trash my doctors and their protocols. She didn't tell me that if I came to Boston and did an IVF cycle at Brigham and Women's I would get a different result.

Rather, she studied my records, thought deeply about my situation, and shared with me her clear-eyed view of my case, the landscape of infertility treatment, and what I could and should be looking for in my next doctor if I wanted to keep trying. Essentially, she taught me how to look at fertility specialists and clinics more critically with respect to what they could offer me, as an individual, as opposed to generalized statistics. It may sound subtle, but this shift in thinking is, in my view, the primary reason that I was ultimately able to succeed.

We reviewed my previous IVF protocols together, and while certainly not cutting-edge, Rachel found them to be reasonable, and not too different from what she would have prescribed, except for the time of transfer, where she strongly favored waiting until the embryo was three or five days old, rather than two, giving it more time to develop. She pointed out that most other good clinics would follow a similar protocol, perhaps tinkering at the margins. But more important, she also told me that new research and new treatments were evolving in other countries and in certain places in the United States, and that if I was determined to keep trying, I might want to consider those. She instinctively felt that my miscarriages and IVF failures most likely resulted from aneuploidy. Aneuploidy, Rachel explained, was simply an abnormal number of chromosomes in a cell, meaning a cell either had an extra chromosome (trisomy) or was missing one (monosomy) instead of having the normal pair. With the exception of a few specific abnormalities, such as trisomy 21, which results in Down syndrome, most embryos with aneuploid cells are not compatible with life and are miscarried.

Although not offered at Brigham and Women's at that time, Rachel explained that there was a relatively new technology called preimplantation genetic screening (PGS)[2] in which a cell was removed from a three-day-old embryo (created through IVF) and assessed for common chromosomal abnormalities by testing five to seven pairs of chromosomes. Only embryos deemed to be normal were transferred to the womb. It was too early to conclusively evaluate the success of PGS, but doctors were publishing results that looked promising, and in light of what she suspected were my repeat aneuploid embryos, Rachel felt that in my case it might make sense to explore. She jotted down some names of people in New York and Europe for me to look up.

We also discussed the topic of reproductive immunology treatment, which, like PGS, was not offered at Brigham and Women's. Because it required suppressing the immune system, Rachel did not support that particular treatment—she felt there was not enough evidence of efficacy to countermand the risks—but she told me where to go to look for more information to educate myself.

I left her office feeling overwhelmed but also energized. There was so much more to learn. There were new things I could try. I was thirty-six, and I had to hurry, but my journey was not over.

I needed to know more about the quality of my embryos. Although still in its infancy and not yet mainstream in either the United Kingdom or the United States, I discovered that PGS was available at a half-dozen clinics, several of which had very high success rates, and in our case, after four miscarriages, I believed it was essential.

I also needed to learn more about my own immunological system. Was it possible that my immune system itself was causing the miscarriages, my own natural killer cells attacking our fetus as it would a foreign body?

The information I sought was not all to be found locally. I pondered the immunity question with the sympathetic wife of a client of mine, who was keeping a watchful eye on my fertility travails. She had urged me to see her doctor in Geneva for a second opinion when I was diagnosed with antiphospholipid syndrome, which I did, and now she absolutely insisted that I go to Frankfurt to see a doctor widely known for his expertise in this particular area. Not accustomed to taking no for an answer, my fertility fairy godmother arranged it all. I flew to Frankfurt, was met by a driver and translator, and whisked off to the medical campus of the University of Frankfurt, where in a one-hour meeting, one of the world's leading scientists researching natural killer cells gave me my next medical directions: during my subsequent IVF cycle, for which he strongly urged PGS, I would suppress my immune system with intravenous immuno-globulin, or IVIG, to prevent it from potentially harming an embryo.

Taking it all in, I felt grateful then, and many times since, that my often-too-demanding job had led to this unexpected side benefit, open-ing doors to doctors and practices that I would not otherwise know about, let alone have the capability to access. For the first time in my medically assisted quest to have a baby, I felt empowered rather than timidly led along.

Returning to London, I optimistically prepared for my next IVF cycle at the highly regarded Lister Fertility Clinic in London (chosen after much research and consultation) with a great new team and a new protocol, which was to include:

- A different level and combination of hormones to stimulate my eggs to grow [3]
- Viagra to thicken my uterine lining in an effort to increase the odds of implantation [4]
- Intracytoplasmic sperm injection (ICSI)—in which a sperm is injected directly into an egg in an effort to encourage

fertilization—to half of my eggs to test whether, despite no
indication of male factor infertility, this would improve our
fertilization rate (it had no effect)
- IVIG to convince my immune system that our tiny embryo was
  not a hostile foreigner
- Genetic testing through PGS to select chromosomally normal
  embryos.

One of the reasons I had chosen the Lister for treatment was its
ability to do PGS. Our plan was to test all our embryos on day three,
and to transfer two normal blastocysts—ideally evolved from the embryos by the time the testing is complete—to my uterus two days later.

To my great surprise, when I went for a baseline blood test often
administered before an IVF cycle commences, I discovered that I was
pregnant again, naturally. This time I knew well enough not to get my
hopes up, and I was smart not to do so. Despite heparin shots and IVIG
transfusions to combat my blood clots and suppress my overactive immune system, my fifth pregnancy led to my fifth miscarriage, confirmed
at St. Mary's Hospital on a date I will never forget, as it was the same day
as the devastating 7/7 London bombing. As I sat in the hospital waiting
room for agonizing hours, listening as news about the attack trickled
in, I was joined by a steady stream of injured victims. They stumbled
through the doors, some bloody, some limping, some clenched in pain,
some visibly in shock. By the end of the day, more than fifty people had
died and hundreds were injured. Surrounded by survivors, I was forced
to confront tragedies greater than my own.

The fifth miscarriage didn't devastate me the way the others had. I
was beyond emotions now. My resolve only strengthened: I would succeed. It was the only way to be able to handle the previous losses. We
would try IVF again armed with all our newfound knowledge about fertility treatments: fertilization with ICSI; genetic testing of our embryos,
which we would grow to day five blastocysts; Viagra; blood thinners;
immune suppression; progesterone support; acupuncture; nutritional

and hormone supplements. We would leave no stone unturned. We would eliminate all chance of miscarriage again.

And maybe we would have. It is hard to know. Because despite our collective efforts—and my doctors at this clinic were truly heroic trying everything they could throughout two more cycles—I did not get pregnant again through conventional IVF.

Like me, Jessica took charge of her fertility following a terrible scare. After multiple IVF cycles, multiple pregnancies, and multiple miscarriages as a well-informed but relatively passive patient, Jessica's clinic required her to undergo yet another hysterosalpingogram (HSG), despite her objections to repeating this diagnostic test to assess the anatomical structure of the uterus. After the invasive procedure, performed on her as an outpatient, Jessica experienced extreme and continuous bleeding. She called her clinic several times that afternoon, increasingly panicked each time, but did not elicit much concern from the nurses, who merely asked how many pads she was bleeding through per hour. Finally, her husband, Ethan, a physician, called the clinic and told the nurses that Jessica was bleeding through one hundred pads in a thirty-minute time frame. He rushed her to the hospital emergency room, where doctors, discovering her uterus had been nicked in the procedure, had to cauterize and then stitch her to control the bleeding. The emergency room team saved her life. In the depths of her despair, Jessica decided two things: she wanted an apology (which never came), and she was going to take charge of her fertility.

When Marcy, much to her surprise, was diagnosed with low ovarian reserve at age thirty-two, she and her husband, Dan, were told that they would face an uphill battle conceiving a child. As Marcy and Dan, both lawyers, processed the shocking news that she had far fewer eggs left than a typical woman of her age, potentially of lower quality as well, they determined to approach infertility treatments with a critical eye, rapidly educating themselves about the available procedures and statistics. Yet despite all the information they collected, as they attempted to navigate the largely unfamiliar world of infertility, they generally deferred to the advice of the experts. When Marcy was rushed to the hospital in the seventh month of her pregnancy, they tragically learned that the experts are not always right. Unwilling to heed their pleas to wait for Marcy's fertility doctor to arrive, the emergency room doctors proceeded with a plan to operate on Marcy despite her objections. Her baby's heartbeat stopped during surgery. After losing her beloved baby at twenty-six weeks, Marcy suddenly understood: "I am the only person who will advocate for myself. I have to step up and take responsibility."

Taking control of one's fertility starts, to some degree, with ensuring that you are at the right clinic. But a great many women (myself included) choose their clinic—at least their first clinic—based on convenience or a referral from their ob-gyn. "Think of the care a couple might put into choosing a car or washing machine, yet for something as monumental as where they are going to have their IVF treatment they don't ask the clinic any questions. They just go where a friend went," noted the director of a fertility clinic.[5]

Success rates for different age groups and conditions vary dramatically, not only around the world, but also within a city, state, or country, and it is imperative to find the best clinic available for you. The only way to do so is to be armed with the right questions.

I realize that it may seem that I moved around and switched clinics an awful lot—two fertility clinics in London, one in New York, and eventually one in Moscow, with consultations in Boston, Geneva, and Frankfurt. While the far-flung array of cities I frequented may be unique, clinic shopping is certainly not. In fact, most fertility patients will leave their first doctor.[6] Paula began her fertility treatments consulting with one of the nation's leading experts at a top clinic in Colorado. After her first miscarriage and four failed IUI attempts, she switched to another doctor at the same clinic. Following an unsuccessful try with IVF, she sought out a clinic with a doctor who specialized in working with older women. She got pregnant there, but suffered another miscarriage.

When she eventually decided to use a donor egg, she went back to the first clinic. Later, upon learning of her immunology issues, she went to a renowned center in Chicago that offered specialized treatments.

Sarah, from Massachusetts, similarly sought out a famous clinic in Manhattan after repeated failures in Boston; unimpressed, she continued treatment with her Boston clinic. Rose, a teacher who had to terminate her first pregnancy due to the diagnosis of her baby's fatal brain malformation, left her first clinic after multiple tries, frustrated and feeling that the doctors there were simply following a standard protocol that didn't make sense for her. "They had just two protocols," she told me angrily, "that's it. They don't individualize." She interviewed two new fertility clinics with outstanding success rates, and chose the one with the doctor with whom she felt more comfortable, and who offered a more personalized treatment plan.

Anna, the social worker, started out in her hometown of Denver at a clinic with success rates among the highest in the country; she left it when she felt the doctors were unwilling, or perhaps not able, to tailor treatment to accommodate her lupus, an autoimmune problem. She sought out a clinic in Chicago that specialized in reproductive immunology, hoping to combine the recommended immune therapies with IVF at her Denver clinic. "She basically laughed in my face," Anna recounted when telling me about her original fertility doctor. "I felt like she was saying, 'You don't know anything; we know everything.' It was almost like they were insulted." Anna turned to a different clinic in Denver with a doctor who was more than happy to work with her immunologist. "They were in so much communication, it was amazing," she happily recalled. Anna had her daughter on their first try.

Danielle left her local British clinic after three failed attempts and sought out a famously controversial doctor with the highest success rates in London after her husband found him through his research. My good friend Susan in London left the Lister, where she had once had great confidence, opting to try a famous doctor in New York.

Everyone is going every which way.

Is there rhyme or reason to it?

Certain clinics, often with high success rates, are lightning rods. As in every industry, there are outliers—those who achieve success far greater than the norm. In the case of fertility, their approaches and practices are routinely called into question. Are they turning away difficult cases? Taking unnecessary risks, such as implanting high numbers of embryos? Throwing "the kitchen sink" at patients, regardless of clear need or even of the health of the patient? Or are they genuinely superior? These questions are very hard to answer, and it seems that for each patient running to a famous doctor, there is another running away at equal speed. Ironically, in the same week, one woman I interviewed called her doctor a god, and another told me that she had just run into that very same doctor at a restaurant and the sight of him made her so upset and angry that she couldn't eat her meal.

Scientific and technological advances have given doctors—and patients—a bigger tool kit with which to treat previously insurmountable problems. But with great advances in medicine comes a great mass of information to sort through. What works? What doesn't? How does a patient decide? How much does the practitioner matter? How does a patient choose a clinic? As I learned during my journey, this new world of fertility is complex and changing, and patients must be educated and involved in order to successfully navigate through it.

In my view, when deciding whether and where to do IVF, it is wise to evaluate certain key treatment elements that are critical, if not essential, differentiators among clinics, apart from the (often obscure) measure of their success rates. These elements are: tailored drug protocols, blastocyst capabilities, and availability and sophistication of genetic screening.

Protocols

The first stage in any IVF cycle involves preparing a woman's ovaries to produce one or more eggs to be retrieved and then fertilized before being placed back into the womb. In all but a natural cycle (the rarest form of IVF), a woman takes a series of drugs intended to stimulate, in most cases, the greatest number of eggs for removal. While traditional IVF has different regimen options (for example, the GnRH agonist, also known as Lupron downregulation, protocol; the GnRH antagonist, or ganirelix, protocol; the microflare protocol), the general goal of each phase remains consistent: women take hormones to stimulate the growth of eggs, control the timing of ovulation, and prepare the uterus for implantation. Since its inception, there has been remarkably little variation in the protocols. "For nearly thirty years we've been doing the same thing," lamented Dr. Laura Rienzi, senior clinical embryologist and laboratory director of the GENERA Centres for Reproductive Medicine in Italy. "We're just doing what they did at the beginning of IVF, but the physical and chemical environment is so important."[7]

Because no two women are alike, a fertility expert should ideally tailor the cocktail to suit the individual medical situation. There are reasons that one hormone may be preferable to another at any given stage of the process. For example, for the stimulation phase of my cycle, I was first prescribed Puregon (FSH) but switched in subsequent cycles to Menopur (FSH and LH). I later learned that adding LH to the mix was not advisable for patients with PCOS, who already often have abnormally high LH levels. The additional LH placed me at greater risk of hyperstimulation (which, in fact, occurred). Similarly, while the agonist and antagonist protocols are used in fairly equal numbers among fertility clinics, women with repeat implantation failure, poor ovarian response to stimulation, and PCOS have been found to experience improved embryo quality and higher implantation and pregnancy rates using the more recently developed antagonist protocol.[8]

In the same vein, most IVF protocols rely on an injection of HCG thirty-six hours prior to egg collection to trigger ovulation. Like the vast majority of IVF patients, I took the HCG trigger shot in all my IVF cycles. But the HCG shot lingers in the body for ten days, continuing to support hormone production in the ovaries, risking hyperstimulation.

Moreover, the standard dosage of ten thousand units originally came from veterinary medicine, and may in fact be too high for most women, or at least higher than they need to be effective. Experts believe that a dosage of only half that amount does the trick at less risk to the growing eggs of the patient. Although far less commonly prescribed, some specialists are now swapping out the HCG altogether in favor of Lupron, or using Lupron in combination with lower amounts of HCG, which they believe can get the ovulation job done with virtually no risk of OHSS.[9] While the ten-thousand-unit trigger has been the gold standard for decades, it is important to look at the pros and cons of the newer options for each particular patient.

These choices matter, and can make the difference between having a baby and not having a baby. Danielle and her husband credit their beautiful four-year-old twins, born after years of failure, to the famously obsessive daily tweaking of her protocol by a doctor who she felt "was on top of every single aspect of [her] health and care." IVF protocols are constantly evolving, and the ever-increasing knowledge is resulting in greater and greater success. But not all clinics are keeping up, and not all doctors are cognizant of the changes, as well as the important impact of subtle tweaking of protocols. It is critically important to ask your doctor detailed questions about your protocol and why he or she believes it is the best for you.

Blastocysts

A blastocyst is to an embryo kind of like a teenager is to an infant. That is, you can tell a lot more about what kind of being it will grow up to be as it matures. An embryo starts out as a single-cell organism inside a protective shell. The cell separates into two cells within the first twenty-four hours, then the two into four, and ideally, four into eight. Although the rate of cell division varies, typically, on day three, a healthy embryo will have around eight cells. Up to this point, the embryo's growth is fueled by its mother's egg, much as an infant is dependent on its mother's milk. But in order to survive past this stage, the embryo must activate its own genes to propel its development. By day four, a thriving embryo will have between sixteen and thirty-two cells, at which point it is called a morula. In the next one to two days, the morula undergoes a huge growth spurt in which a fluid-filled cavity forms in its center, the cells keep dividing into two hundred to three hundred cells, and differentiation of the embryo begins. This far more complex version of the embryo is called a blastocyst. Not all embryos are capable of making this difficult transition to independence. In fact, only about one-third of all normal-looking embryos successfully evolve into blastocysts. Yet these survivors are healthier, stronger, and more highly developed than the rest of the pack. As a result, they have a greater chance of growing into fetuses, and eventually, healthy children.

From the early days of IVF (including my first two cycles with Mr. P), nascent four-cell embryos were transferred on the second day after their creation in the lab (day two). The procedure then evolved into doing transfers at day three, at which stage the clinicians had more observable information about the embryos, as they could see which had developed into eight-cell embryos, and speculate from their appearance as to which of those would be more likely to continue healthy growth. The practice evolved this way due to both technological limitations (early laboratory culture media could only sustain life in the petri dish for two to three days) and a belief, now dispelled, that the embryos were more likely to thrive in the womb than in the lab.[10] Because it is difficult at best to predict with accuracy on day two or day three which embryos are more likely to produce a viable pregnancy, multiple embryos are often transferred.

Yet, biologically, transferring an embryo to the uterus on day two or day three is earlier than what occurs in a natural conception, in which an embryo at this stage would still be growing in the fallopian tube. A naturally created embryo would typically arrive in the uterus five or six days after conception, precisely when it would be ready to hatch and the endometrium would be ready to receive it. Improvements in the culture medium now enable embryos to grow to the blastocyst stage, leading not only to a more informed selection of healthy embryos but also facilitating the transfer of these embryos at the optimal time for implantation in the womb. Importantly, improved selection of viable embryos with a greater chance of success means that far fewer, and ideally only one embryo can be transferred to the mother, reducing the risk of pregnancy complications and multiple births.

The success rates certainly bear out the theory, with some clinics reporting pregnancy and live birth rates of day five blastocyst transfers that more than double the rates of day three embryo transfers. Notably, the differential tends to increase with age, with women aged forty-one and forty-two experiencing an almost 150 percent increase in live birth rates when transferring blastocysts.[11]

Challengingly, blastocysts can be hard to come by. By the time Sarah and Evan learned of her clotting disorder, they had experienced four losses and wanted to do everything in their power to avoid another nightmarish *Groundhog Day*. For their next cycle, in addition to Sarah's immune therapies, they were planning to try a blastocyst transfer. Accustomed to bountiful egg harvests, they weren't particularly concerned about their numbers, but it was nerve-racking to see Sarah's fifteen eggs dwindle down to just four blastocysts, only one of which was ultimately viable.

Anna, the social worker who underwent immune treatments for her lupus, had a nail-biter as well. Anna produced five eggs, three of which fertilized, and she knew that with those odds her chances were slim. As it turned out, her three embryos resulted in exactly one normal blastocyst, as bookies would predict.

During my first two IVF cycles, I had produced not only copious amounts of eggs but also enjoyed a large number of beautiful (round, nonfragmented) grade I and II embryos. Sixteen eggs obtained in the first cycle yielded twelve embryos, seven of which were deemed to be high quality on day two, while twenty-six eggs obtained in the second cycle led to nineteen embryos, twelve of which were deemed to be of similarly high quality. Mr. P frequently commented about my being a great producer of gorgeous embryos, focusing his efforts on making the embryos stick.

My cycle at the Lister started out much like the others. I had twenty-four eggs, nineteen of which developed into embryos. Given the large pool, the clinic immediately froze eight embryos for a potential future frozen embryo transfer—for a sibling, they explained, optimistic of success. We kept the remaining fertilized batch of embryos in the lab for four more days, planning to transfer two blastocysts on day five. Each doctor we spoke with warned us about the risk of multiples, especially as blastocysts had a far higher rate of implantation, but we weren't daunted. After our failures and frustration, two seemed like a good deal. We never had to make that final decision though. When we arrived at the clinic bright and early for the much-anticipated transfer, we learned that only one normal blastocyst had made it that far. But it was absolutely flawless, the doctor and embryologist assured us. A winner.

Sadly, this picture-perfect blastocyst did not successfully take up residence in my womb.

Preimplantation Genetic Diagnosis (PGD) and Screening (PGS)

The reality is that we just can't learn very much about the health and viability of an embryo by simply looking at it. If only I had a dollar for every woman I spoke with who told me about her amazing A / A+ / A++ / grade I / grade II embryos that unfortunately did not bring the dearly hoped-for baby. Fortunately, although many embryos are still selected that way throughout the IVF world, doctors and patients no longer need be dependent on the human eye alone.

Progress in the field of genetic testing of embryos formed in vitro is perhaps one of the most exciting and promising developments in the field of treating infertility, and it has been a long time coming. Dr. John Rock, who fertilized the first human egg in a glass test tube in his lab at Harvard in 1944, predicted back in 1937 not only that human babies would be born of embryos created in labs but also that one day science would enable parents to choose to have a son or daughter.[12] More than fifty years after Dr. Rock's prediction, in 1990, the first baby girls were born as a result of IVF performed using preimplantation genetic diagnosis (PGD), testing the pair of sex chromosomes in a single cell removed from the embryo in order to select females, XX, rather than males, XY. The genetic testing enabled the parents to eliminate the risk of their children being born with adrenoleukodystrophy and mental retardation, genetic diseases typically affecting only males.[13]

PGD, which tests one chromosome for a specific genetic disease, grew from gender testing to include a wide array of abnormalities linked to single genes, such as cystic fibrosis, and inherited blood disorders, like sickle cell disease.[14] Just under two years after the first successful PGD birth, the same team helped a couple who were genetic carriers of cystic fibrosis to have a normal girl unaffected by cystic fibrosis and free of both parents' genetic mutation.[15] Detection of a mutation in an embryo's DNA enabled clinicians to weed them out. The early technology was relatively slow, requiring weeks or months of work by highly skilled scientists, with a typical waiting period of three to six months to obtain results. Within the last five years, however, rapid progress has led to a new process called karyomapping, capable of accurately identifying all single-gene disorders, generally in as little as two to four weeks. As a result of karyomapping, according to Dr. Mark Hughes, a molecular biochemist who was one of the founding fathers of PGD, "there are no technical limitations anymore for inherited disorders."[16] Just think about that. Genetic mutations like those that cause cystic fibrosis and Tay-Sachs can now—given the directive and resources—be completely eliminated. A mother with breast cancer can prevent her offspring from inheriting her BRCA1 mutation.[17]

PGD's success in detecting specific disorders led scientists on a quest to test more chromosomes, looking not to identify a specific inherited disease but rather to identify embryos with too few or too many chromosomes, which would render them impaired or incapable of survival—and which is the most common cause of failed pregnancies. To their surprise, they found that *lethal* chromosome defects were detected in the lab in seemingly normal chromosomes.[18] Simply put, we cannot see chromosomal abnormalities with the human eye. As a result, in an effort to help doctors and patients select chromosomally normal embryos most capable of progressing through a healthy pregnancy, preimplantation genetic screening (PGS), also known as aneuploidy screening, was born.

While it took fifty-three years for Dr. Rock's prediction of sex selection to come true, scientific advances in the last five to ten years are moving at breakneck speed. When I first tried PGS, in 2005, my clinic used a technique called fluorescence in situ hybridization, or FISH, testing. The first available technology for PGS, and for nearly two decades the gold standard, FISH typically screened the seven chromosomes most frequently seen in miscarriage specimens (chromosomes 13, 16, 18, 21, 22, X, and Y). The embryologist would remove one cell from each day three embryo (having ideally eight cells, but embryos with five to nine cells might be tested), analyze the specified chromosomes in the selected cells, and within forty-eight hours, transfer the embryos deemed to be normal, if any, back to the mother.

Although theoretically an unequivocal improvement, PGS has been highly controversial, primarily for two reasons. First, given the relative youth and instability of the three-day-old embryos, doctors legitimately feared that healthy embryos could be lost or destabilized during the biopsy process—a concern that was reinforced by early studies revealing lower pregnancy rates and live birth rates among women who used PGS.[19] In addition, both critics and supporters alike discovered another challenge to successful genetic testing—a phenomenon called mosaicism.

In a perfect embryo, the genetic makeup of all cells in the embryo is identical. A mosaic embryo is one in which not all of its cells are genetically the same; some cells might be chromosomally normal and others abnormal. Although all derived from a single cell, errors can occur during the repeated cell divisions, leaving an intended pairing with too many or too few chromosomes. A single-cell biopsy renders only one set of data points and might not be reflective of the whole embryo. Mosaicism, therefore, could lead to both false positives and false negatives; that is, the tested cell could be normal, while others in the embryo were abnormal, meaning a "bad egg" could be transferred, or conversely, the tested specimen might be the sole, or one of the few abnormal cells, and an otherwise healthy egg might be inadvertently discarded.

Perhaps surprisingly, unlike chromosomal abnormalities, mosaicism is not at all correlated to maternal age. Women over forty-two do not have higher rates of mosaics than women under thirty-five.[20] Experts believe that this is likely explained by the fact that mosaicism results from a mitotic cell division after the embryo is formed, as opposed to meiotic errors present in the egg of the mother, known to be correlated with age.[21]

It is literally jaw-dropping how far the technology has developed in the decade since I first tried PGS. A single cell of a human embryo has twenty-three pairs of chromosomes (twenty-two pairs of nonsex chromosomes, plus the X and Y pairing). The FISH method was capable of testing eleven data points, essentially one cell on each of eleven chromosomes, although many clinics tested only five, seven, or nine chromosomes. The next "gold standard" of testing, array comparative genomic hybridization (aCGH), which came on the IVF scene in the mid to late 2000s and is still used in many clinics today, tested *twenty-seven hundred data points on all twenty-four chromosomes*, detecting far more abnormalities than FISH had been capable of detecting.[22] Yet despite its remarkable improvements in detecting abnormalities, like its predecessor, aCGH could not detect mosaic embryos.

The newest technology, high-resolution next generation sequencing (NGS or hrNGS), produced its first baby in 2013, and has become more readily available in the last few years. Also known as PGS 2.0, high-resolution NGS is capable of testing *1.2 million data points*, and for the first time, identifying mosaic embryos. Use of high-resolution NGS has also illuminated the size of the mosaicism problem, which may represent as many as 20 percent of all embryos produced in the lab.[23] In fact, NGS can see mosaicism so precisely that genetics labs can now tell patients exactly what percent of mosaicism is present in a given embryo, with far-reaching implications for pregnancy and live birth rates. For example, an embryo judged to be normal using aCGH was transferred to a woman who became pregnant and subsequently lost the baby at seven weeks. The recovered fetal tissue was subjected to NGS, which revealed a trisomy on chromosome 4, a mutation that would have been detected with preimplantation NGS.[24] As a result of this enhanced analysis, miscarriage rates are cut in half when using high-resolution NGS as opposed to aCGH.[25]

Hand in hand with the development of NGS technology has been the ability to test multiple cells from the outer shell of more robust day five blastocysts as opposed to a single cell from a day three embryo, largely eradicating the fear of harming the embryo. Moreover, because blastocysts are more developed, they are also less likely to be abnormal or mosaic—as abnormals are less likely to make it to day five—and are able to contribute more DNA for testing. The ability to select embryos based upon such extensive knowledge of their chromosomal makeup has important implications, including transferring fewer embryos per cycle, and in many cases a single blastocyst.

While not a first choice for embryo selection, mosaicism is not necessarily a death knell. Rather, it is a calculated risk. Many healthy babies have been born from mosaic embryos. A study in Italy in 2015 found that six out of eighteen women who had abnormal embryos transferred to their womb gave birth to healthy children.[26] Dr. Santiago Munné, cofounder of Reprogenetics[27]—the world's largest genetics laboratory specializing in PGD and PGS—led a multicenter study that reported 58 successful pregnancies out of 143 mosaic transfers, and Dr. Munné believes that more than one hundred babies have been born of mosaic embryos so far.[28] How can this be? Scientists theorize that the embryos may have the ability to self-heal, essentially ejecting the abnormal cells while the normal cells continue to divide.[29]

Yet Dr. Munné and his colleague Dr. Dagan Wells of the University of Oxford emphasize that mosaic blastocysts, while capable of producing healthy babies, do not fare as well overall as normal embryos, implanting significantly less frequently and miscarrying three times more often.[30] Moreover, they contend, all mosaics are not created equal; some embryos have only single or minimal aberrations, while others have complex abnormalities. Based on persuasive data made possible by hrNGS testing, Munné, Wells, and a society of experts believe it is time for a new classification system, with low-level mosaics (less than 20 percent abnormal cells) being treated as normal; high-level (greater than 80 percent abnormal cells) mosaics labeled as aneuploid; and a new, third category (those with 20 to 80 percent abnormal cells) classified as "mosaic" embryos, distinct from their normal (euploid) and abnormal (aneuploid) brethren.[31] Determining what level is safe and prudent to transfer is gray, and not surprisingly, a subject of debate among fertility experts. However, recognizing the possibility that some of the lower-level mosaics may be capable of survival, in May 2017, a committee of the American Society for Reproductive Medicine declared transfer of these mosaics to be "ethically permissible."

The bottom line: despite a risk of miscarriage, in the absence of any normal embryos, transfer of a low-level mosaic may present a woman's best, in fact only, chance of success.

The results of preimplantation genetic screening performed using the new high-resolution NGS technology are hard to argue with, although there are, of course, still PGS detractors. There are undoubtedly those who, faced with the quandary of mosaics, sympathize with those who might believe that "perhaps the best advance now for IVF is to take a step backward" and transfer embryos without testing them.[32] Yet randomized clinical trials, meta-analyses, the Centers for Disease Control and Prevention, and fertility clinics all agree: embryos subjected to PGS have demonstrably higher success rates.[33,34,35] One study showed a near doubling in the live birth rate for women under thirty-four years old using hrNGS, a tripling for women aged thirty-eight to forty, and *a tenfold increase* for women aged forty-one to forty-two, while the overall miscarriage rate fell from 50 percent to 14 percent. Remarkably, the women in the PGS group transferred fewer embryos per cycle—in most cases only a single blastocyst—and saw an average increase of 97 percent in live birth rates per first transfer attempt.[36]

Additionally, of great significance for women worried about their age—an increasingly large group these days—PGS eliminates any maternal age effect on implantation rates.[37] In one study, women aged forty-one and forty-two had implantation rates of more than 70 percent, higher than those of women under forty. Women without PGS, in contrast, saw implantation rates drop from 40 percent among those under thirty-five, to less than 5 percent among those over forty-two.[38] On top of that, the miscarriage rate among women utilizing PGS does not increase with maternal age, in stark contrast with greatly heightened pregnancy loss—from approximately 10 percent for women under thirty-five to over 50 percent among women over forty-two—among those who do not have PGS.[39]

Accurate PGS is the great equalizer. If the embryo is chromosomally normal, odds are it will implant and survive.

FISH was first-generation technology; the equivalent of the dial-up telephone. And now with hrNGS we have the smartphone version. With previously unimaginable results: Fewer embryos transferred. Low risk of multiples. Reduced risk of miscarriage. Diminished impact of age. It's a game changer, if you have the right technology and the right operator.

Unfortunately, many clinics are still using earlier generation technologies that are missing a lot of the diagnoses, particularly the mosaics.

These clinics achieve the be-all-and-end-all high pregnancy rates so sought after in the field, but if they tracked their patients, experts believe they would also report high miscarriage rates.[40]

Yet even the dial-up version was enough to convince me. My first foray with PGS at the Lister clearly demonstrated how little could be ascertained about the viability of my embryos by just looking at them. Although my doctor warned me that testing the embryos could potentially harm them, it seemed worth the risk to me. With eleven embryos to test (and eight more in the freezer), I did not feel overly concerned about losing a few. When we received a call informing us that only one was normal, I was shocked by the result. We went from *twenty-four* eggs to *one* normal blastocyst.

I was starting to understand just how stacked the odds were against me.

All sorrows can be borne if you put them into
a story or tell a story about them.

Isak Dinesen

8

The Dark Horse

The Silent Faces of Miscarriage

I *dreaded* calling my mother to tell her about my fifth miscarriage. I
knew she would be devastated, and I feared it would be awkward as
I had not yet told her that I was pregnant.

"Is there something else you're not telling me?" my mother asked as
delicately as she could after I delivered the news. I'm sure she was afraid
of setting me off.

"No. Why?"

"Because you sound energized. Almost cheerful."

I don't think I realized, until hearing her puzzled (and undoubtedly
concerned) voice on the phone, how much my reaction to my latest
miscarriage differed from my earlier reactions—and from the reaction
one would normally expect from a woman who had just lost her fifth
baby. This time, I was beyond the grief and despair that had consumed

me with each previous miscarriage; I was focusing solely on my future success.

But now the memory and the pain of my first miscarriage came back to me, as though I were still sitting in Dr. Simona's office at the Fetal Medicine Centre staring intently at the monitor, which looked a bit like an old-fashioned black-and-white TV. My teary eyes had tried to focus as I sought to make sense of the still image on the screen. I couldn't look at Dr. Simona and the nurse, standing silently by my side. I knew what was happening, and I knew I would not be able to keep it together.

Lost in thought with my mother still waiting on the phone, I realized that my body had assumed my statue-like demeanor, almost bracing myself for the words that were to come. Whether she felt I'd had enough time, or wasn't sure I understood what was happening, or simply had to move on to her next patient, Dr. Simona had broken the silence:

"Unfortunately, there is no heartbeat. The fetus is not viable."

With her words, my world fell apart.

For as often as miscarriages happen, they often remain shrouded in mystery. What causes a miscarriage? Is it preventable? How often does it occur? Why did this happen to me? Was it the coffee? Did I exercise too much? Did we have sex too much? Could I have done something differently?

For most people who have experienced miscarriage, the questions never stop.

Frustratingly, the medical answers can be hard to come by, often because no answers exist. Yet the loss is as much an emotional experience as it is a physical one, and in this respect, there are some things I've come to know about miscarriage.

The Reality of Miscarriage

Miscarriage is devastating. Particularly so when it has been a challenge to conceive. Whether at four days, four weeks, or four months into a pregnancy, the life inside exists no more. It can be hard for those who have not suffered through it, my former self included, to fully comprehend that basic fact: miscarriage is the loss of a life.

A research team at Imperial College London found that *nearly half* of all women who suffered a miscarriage experience symptoms of posttraumatic stress disorder at the time and shortly after the loss, and that four out of ten women continue to report post-traumatic stress months later.[1] Although rarely talked about, having a miscarriage is an experience most women never forget.

It is also, very often, shocking. Especially a first miscarriage. Prior to the moment that I rushed to the ladies' room in my law firm's office in London, nearly doubled over with cramps, desperately hoping I was wrong, and frantically discovered blood in my underwear, I, like almost every other woman I've met who has miscarried, rarely thought or talked about miscarriage. There is no way to prepare either physically or emotionally for miscarriage when it is not even in your field of vision.

"I had a bathroom-floor-on-hands-and-knees moment. Those moments are real," recalls Jessica. Jessica and Ethan were fortunate to have experienced relatively smooth success when they turned to assisted reproductive technology to help them conceive their first child. They were optimistic that they would conceive again fairly easily when they decided to try for a sibling. And they did. But to their shock, they learned at the first ultrasound that the fetus didn't look good. They were told to come back in a week. After an agonizingly slow seven days of praying for the best and fearing the worst, they returned to the clinic hand in hand, where they were informed that their baby had not survived. "It was so much harder mentally and emotionally than physically," Jessica recounts.

That week of waiting. There are no words to describe the agony. I had been there too, as have so many others. You exist in a state in which you truly feel adrift. You realize you are at work, but have no idea how you got there. No idea how you got dressed that morning. No memory of what you ate, where you've been, or what you've said. Your only thought is of that baby in your womb, and whether it is alive.

Paula remembers this period as "hell." Her doctor told her at her first ultrasound scan that there was a 98 percent chance of her miscarrying, and, like Jessica, that she should come back in a week. Sadly, her doctor was right. Her second pregnancy was the same. And the third. She and her husband, Derrick, saw the fetus and the heartbeat at the first ultrasound, and it was all over by the next. By the third miscarriage, they were in such despair that Derrick sank to his knees and screamed.

Sarah and Evan similarly experienced agonizing waits and terrifying ultrasounds with each of Sarah's four miscarriages. Since they had never made it past two ultrasounds without being met by disaster, and were conditioned to expect the worst, Sarah describes her first trimesters as "brutal." "Our hearts were palpitating at each scan," she told me. "We had so many that our refrigerator was covered in them," Evan added.

Jessica became so obsessed with becoming pregnant that the minute she was physically able, she started trying again. IVF stimulation drugs. Embryo transfer. Positive pregnancy test. Troubling ultrasound scan. No heartbeat. Repeat. With each miscarriage, the shock dissipated, but the sadness set in for the long term. She and her husband developed coping skills to get through the toughest times. Jessica needed time on her own to grieve, but Ethan preferred to lean in and be together. They found their balance. She would go on long walks and then return to him. "As you go through life," Jessica reflects, "you redefine your normal."

Of course, no time is an especially good time to lose a baby, but, in my experience, miscarriages tend to come at particularly inconvenient moments. My first began shortly after I had started working in the London office, while I was meeting with my new boss. My third started en route to a friend's birthday dinner. To this day I don't know why or how I did it, but I somehow managed to smile and get through the party without letting anybody know, including my husband. My fourth miscarriage happened at an ice polo tournament that should have been the treat of a lifetime. As the spectacular polo ponies in luscious shades of chocolate flew onto the blindingly white ice, impeccably framed by snow-capped mountains and a cerulean sky, I sat in the stands, praying that I wasn't losing my future child. My fifth loss was on the day of the tragic London bombing. And my last miscarriage occurred during a nearly all-male, terribly formal board meeting when I was suddenly overcome with painful and extremely worrying cramping. By then, I knew instantly what the cramps meant and would have liked to run to the bathroom to confirm my worst fears. Instead, I forced myself to sit in the straight-backed chair, feigning interest, while wildly trying to devise a plan to get myself out of that room.

I thought I lived under a black cloud of timing. But it's not just me.

Jessica had her first miscarriage on Christmas Day.

Paula and Derrick learned of Paula's first miscarriage on Good Friday.

Rose, a thirty-six-year-old teacher, and her husband, Mike, learned that their precious fifteen-week-old fetus was not viable on the Fourth of July, with no experienced doctor in sight to perform a necessary medical procedure.

Miscarriage feels lonely, but it is common. Even more so among the fertility challenged. The next time you walk down a crowded street, or go to a movie, or a restaurant, or a baseball game, look at the women around you and contemplate the fact that one in four of them has likely had a miscarriage. One in four of the women in the office. One in four of the women on the train. The March of Dimes estimates that as many as half of all pregnancies may end in miscarriage, although many of these are believed to occur so early they are not even detected.[2] While precise numbers are difficult to obtain, it is commonly believed that approximately 25 percent of all known pregnancies miscarry.

Miscarriage is murky. Although miscarriage is everywhere, far too many still go unexplained, largely unmentioned and unexplored.

Miscarriage is often silent. My experience of losses spanned two extremes: I either was blissfully unaware that the baby inside me had stopped growing, that its impossibly tiny heart had stopped beating; or I knew with sudden and painful certainty that my baby was gone. For whatever reason, my moments of sudden loss always occurred in situations where I was nearly powerless to act and falling to pieces publicly was neither a desirable nor viable option.

So many women feel such pressure to appear calm and not fall apart in the face of a miscarriage. Why the shame? Why the stigma?

I have wondered if it is perhaps because to treat a miscarriage like a death is to recognize that it was a life? Or because miscarriage is regarded in some way as a failure as a woman? Or does it stem from work or other pressures? Or a perception that others don't want to hear about it, that miscarriage somehow isn't a socially acceptable subject to raise.

There is no societal script for reacting to miscarriage, no Hallmark card to tell someone what to say. Perhaps the inconvenience, the sheer untimeliness, of miscarriage contributes to the stoicism that often accompanies it. Women often can't—or at least feel like they can't—react at the time that it is happening and are forced to bottle up the most extreme emotions; yet later, when they might feel it is "appropriate," the moment is lost. The raw immediacy is gone. We have learned, or forced ourselves, to move on in public, to keep it together. It can be hard to bring up the subject again, particularly when to do so for many is to relive the pain, and to confront the fear of being met with silence.

Given how common miscarriage is, the enormity of the lost communication is tragic, especially in light of how much it can help to discuss the loss—to share, to learn, to regain hope. Sarah, who describes herself as a very private person, was unsure at first about whether she wanted to share her story with me. But as we talked, she became increasingly enthusiastic. "If no one is talking about it, you're just suffering," she concluded. "Alone. For no reason really."

Medical Aspects of Miscarriage

The history of the medical study of miscarriage is peppered with erroneous assumptions that have led to decades of false understandings and ineffective therapies. Surprisingly, even the number of women who experience miscarriage has not been well understood. But scientific understanding of miscarriage is constantly evolving, and while much remains unknown, there are more answers today than ever before.

For example, miscarriage, we now know, occurs as frequently as childbirth. Modern detection techniques have led to a new understanding of miscarriage rates, indicating not only that *half* of all pregnancies fail, but also that 25 percent of women who try to become pregnant likely will have two miscarriages, and that another 12.5 percent will have three.[3] This latter figure is in stark contrast to the oft-cited figure that a mere 1 to 2 percent of women will experience multiple, or recurrent, miscarriages. For the women out there, like myself, who suffer recurrent miscarriage loss, these statistics are of huge significance: You are not alone. Not even in the 1 percent. There are others like you, and most will go on to have healthy children.

Miscarriages broadly fall into two categories: sporadic miscarriages and recurrent miscarriages. Sporadic miscarriages, by far the more common and experienced by a quarter of all women, are believed to result from an isolated occurrence, in most cases a chromosomal abnormality, or occasionally, an aggressive infection or virus. At least half of all miscarriages, in fact, result from one or more chromosomal abnormalities in the fetus, a fact borne out by numerous scientific studies, but itself not yet well understood. If half of all pregnancies end in miscarriage, and half of all miscarriages are a result of chromosomal abnormalities, that means that *one in four* embryos conceived has a chromosomal abnormality.

Recurrent miscarriages, by contrast, are generally defined to be three (or, more recently by some clinicians, two) miscarriages in a row, and are thought to result from chronic, underlying causes, such as hormone imbalances, abnormalities in the shape of the uterus, cervical insufficiency, and immune problems.

Traditional thinking on miscarriage holds that while nothing can be done to prevent sporadic miscarriages, action can be taken to remedy certain causes of recurrent miscarriage. Recent scientific research and new thinking on egg quality, however, may lead to innovative views on both. For example, enhanced PGS techniques enabling those undergoing IVF with PGS to select chromosomally normal embryos dramatically reduce sporadic miscarriage rates, as does improving egg quality. At the same time, but tending toward the opposite direction, newer studies reveal that some common treatment protocols for recurrent miscarriage actually have no demonstrable effect on success.

Sporadic Miscarriage

"There is actually something a lot worse than not getting pregnant, and that's getting pregnant and having a loss," said Dr. Mark Hughes, MD, PhD, to a rapt audience including some of the world's leading fertility specialists at the 2016 ART World Congress in New York City.[4] One of the founding fathers of PGD,[5] Dr. Hughes, a molecular biochemist and head of the Genesis Genetics Institute, has devoted much of his career to helping families elude these avoidable losses. In light of the fact that aneuploidy is the number one cause of miscarriage and failed IVF implantations, the allure of eliminating aneuploidy is easy to see. Emphasizing its promise and directly addressing its earlier limitations, Dr. Hughes proceeded to present research on current PGS methods that demonstrably lower a woman's risk of miscarriage to that of only one-third of their non-PGS peers. The evidence showed that when "normal" embryos implanted, they tended to stick around, and for women and couples with repeated miscarriages, like myself, the promise of transferring chromosomally healthy embryos, less likely to result in loss, is extremely persuasive.[6]

Sitting quietly in the back of the ballroom, I felt myself nodding in violent agreement, gratified to hear a doctor say these words. This was exciting news for a field in which chromosomal abnormalities—which cannot be corrected postconception—eclipse all other forms of miscarriage. Screening out abnormal embryos could prevent so much heartache and pain. Nina, the physician in Boston, certainly shared this view. After three miscarriages and a protracted battle with her insurance company (disappointingly, in one of the most insurance friendly states in the country), she and her husband turned to genetic testing at their own expense for their last IVF cycle. To their overwhelming disappointment, they were told that their only two blastocysts were both abnormal. Despite the heartbreak, Nina told me that "it was so much better than having a miscarriage . . . think of all the time wasted on top of the emotional devastation."

Perhaps because it is considered random and occurs so frequently, sporadic miscarriage is perceived by some in the medical field as both uncorrectable and medically trivial. This perception sadly leads some doctors to treat their patients with a level of care that is not commensurate to the great emotional distress patients feel. Jessica, for example, still gets angry when recalling the callousness of the doctor and nurses at her very expensive clinic, who treated her loss as a statistic and focused immediately on her next cycle. Paula, similarly, remembers that minutes after her miscarriage occurred, while she was still in the depths of despair, she was blithely told such loss was to be expected with older eggs and that she needed an egg donor.

Jane, herself in the medical field, recounts in painful detail her conversation with the nurse who confirmed her miscarriage. When she arrived at the hospital emergency room both in great pain and severe distress, her husband informed the nurse that his wife was twelve weeks pregnant. The nurse replied, without a detectable hint of empathy, "Well, is she twelve weeks pregnant or was she twelve weeks pregnant?" Later, during that same visit, Jane went to the bathroom and discovered that she was already passing the fetus, in the form of plum-size clots.

Cognizant that the fetal tissue could be useful for diagnostic purposes, she mentioned it at the nurses' station on her way back to the examination room. A few minutes later, she heard them joking about who on that shift would have to fish out the contents of the toilet bowl.

Speaking with these and other women about the moments following their miscarriages prompted me to reflect on my own vastly different miscarriage experiences. After my first miscarriage, I had little communication from my doctor, who made no attempt to explain to me why it may have occurred or assuage my fears. When I finally went for my belated D&C, I was sent to the delivery floor of a maternity hospital. The pale yellow walls proudly displayed baby art—infant handprints and footprints, photos of beatific babies—while newborn cries provided the soundtrack to my hospital stay. In contrast, when helping me through a later miscarriage, Mr. Braithwaite kindly scheduled me for a D&C the very next day and booked me into the cardiac ward at a different hospital far from sights and sounds of happy new families. Although in both instances the physical procedure was virtually identical, their emotional impact was decidedly different, a distinction worth noting given that most women who have experienced miscarriage describe the emotional trauma as far more difficult than the physical.

While raising the standard for compassionate care seems like a fairly achievable goal, changing the perception that sporadic miscarriage cannot be prevented may be more challenging. Yet there is reason for optimism, as researchers continue to study aspects of miscarriage in order to understand and address underlying factors. Going one step further than the genetic screening that identifies abnormal embryos, scientists are now starting to focus on egg quality and whether and how it might be improved, leading to the creation of a greater proportion of normal embryos.[7] Although the research is in its early days, improving egg quality is a potential game changer. Since abnormal embryos are the number one cause of sporadic miscarriage, addressing poor egg quality—to date viewed as "incurable"—may be nothing short of miraculous.

Recurrent Miscarriage

Recurrent miscarriage veterans tend to speak their own language.

"Seven: six early, one late, five silent, three D&Cs."

That translates to seven miscarriages, six of which were early, generally meaning before a heartbeat was detected, or perhaps simply meaning first trimester; one was later, indicating that it was both more unusual and more surprising, after the heartbeat was seen and the odds of loss declined severely; five were silent miscarriages, an expression invoked when there has been no actual bleed or loss of the fetus, rather the baby's heart has stopped beating inside the womb and was only detected by ultrasound; and three D&Cs signifies three dilation and curettage procedures to evacuate the products of conception, often performed after a silent miscarriage.

The language continues, ripe with acronyms. "PCOS, APS, high FSH, low AMH . . ." Women who fall through the rabbit hole into the world of recurrent miscarriage often rapidly acquire fluency in this new language as they arm themselves to conquer the obstacles nature has placed in their way.

In contrast with their approach to sporadic miscarriage, fertility specialists have long believed in their ability to combat certain causes of recurrent miscarriage. Fortunately for many, some recurrent miscarriage treatments do in fact have a demonstrable record of success, such as taking aspirin or heparin to thin blood clots, or having surgery to repair an ill-formed uterus. But the various remedies, often offered to couples so desperate to have a healthy pregnancy that they will try almost anything (myself and Richard included), range from the scientifically sound to the speculative to practices that have been proven to be bunk.

Balancing the statistical odds of a treatment working against the hope that you may be one of the lucky ones, no matter how low the odds, is an excruciating task. Presented with any prospect of having a child, many patients opt for treatments with no proven record of success. But what if those treatments may actually be harmful, or expose a mother-to-be to unnecessary risk, or actually lower the odds of success? For example, DES, a synthetic hormone widely prescribed to women in the 1950s and 1960s to prevent miscarriage, was later shown to both increase the risk of miscarriage and to cause devastating health effects in both the mothers who took it and their daughters.[8] Doctors and their patients must look critically at the demonstrable upside versus the real-world costs and risks of experimental treatments. Evaluating the efficacy of any of the treatments, however, can be vexing, as many, if not most, pregnant women who have experienced multiple miscarriages will go on to carry to term with no intervention at all, and the majority of treatment protocols have not been validated with randomized, double-blind studies.

The known and suspected causes of recurrent miscarriage that are generally understood to be susceptible to treatment can be grouped into four major categories: hormone imbalances, including polycystic ovarian syndrome (PCOS); anatomical problems, such as an abnormally shaped uterus or an incompetent cervix; antiphospholipid syndrome and other blood-clotting disorders; and immune problems, most commonly referred to as elevated "natural killer" cells.[9] I had the dubious distinction of falling into every one of the four categories, undergoing treatments for all of them.

Hormone Imbalances / Polycystic Ovarian Syndrome

When I learned from my first doctor in DC that I had polycystic ovaries, not only did I not comprehend the impact that it would have on my efforts to get pregnant, the idea of miscarriage could not have been further from my mind. The doctor never said the word *miscarriage* or connected it to PCOS, nor did the many doctors whom I saw over the next several years.

This omission is startling in light of the fact that the most common abnormality found among women with recurrent miscarriage is the telltale string of pearls along the ovaries—the many tiny cysts rendering the namesake polycystic ovaries.[10] While the cysts present the most visible manifestation, polycystic ovaries and PCOS, the syndrome associated with it, are actually an endocrine disorder. Women with polycystic ovaries often have high levels of testosterone and/or insulin, as well as abnormally high levels of LH in relation to FSH (hormones that are key to ovulation, responsible for triggering the release of a mature egg from its follicle), leading, among other problems, to irregular or absent periods. In addition to conspiring to make pregnancy more difficult to achieve, these hormone imbalances pose a challenge to maintaining a pregnancy. In fact, Professor Lesley Regan, director of the Recurrent Miscarriage Clinic and one of the world's leading miscarriage experts, found a miscarriage rate in women with elevated LH levels that was *five times* the rate of women with normal levels.[11] Further large-scale studies of women with PCOS estimate miscarriage rates of up to 60 percent.[12]

Yet despite uncovering the correlation between PCOS and miscarriage, clinicians and researchers alike have struggled to understand the exact mechanism by which they are connected. Treating women with hormone imbalances is a tricky business, and while drugs like clomiphene citrate (Clomid) and letrozole (Femara) have been effective in varying degrees in helping women with PCOS *get* pregnant, it is not clear that they have the same impact on helping women *stay* pregnant. In the absence of a clear cure, doctors have frequently turned to two additional well-traveled paths to prevent hormonally based recurrent miscarriage: metformin (marketed as Glucophage) and progesterone.

The idea behind using metformin, a drug developed for diabetes, is that it will combat the insulin resistance that often accompanies PCOS. It has been prescribed by doctors for many years to help treat women with PCOS, as well as those with unexplained infertility and recurrent miscarriage, whether or not they were diagnosed with glucose intolerance, despite the fact that large-scale studies indicate that, except for certain cases of women with glucose intolerance, metformin is not effective in ovulation induction and combatting infertility.[13,14] As for combatting miscarriage, however, the results, albeit mixed, are more promising. While some studies have failed to demonstrate any improvement in reducing loss and complications of pregnancy,[15] a number of contradictory trials have in fact shown a marked reduction in early pregnancy loss and preterm labor.[16] In the absence of a prohibition, or any clear guideline at all, many doctors opt to throw metformin into the mix and hope it works. My doctors recommended that I try it throughout many cycles while attempting to conceive, and through two (failed) pregnancies. It didn't work for me, but hopefully it didn't hurt either.

Progesterone, a natural hormone that is essential to maintaining a healthy pregnancy, has long been a go-to in the fertility industry—for PCOS, for unexplained miscarriage, and for a condition called luteal phase deficiency (LPD), itself a point of great controversy in the fertility world. Not only is there wide disagreement about whether luteal phase deficiency exists, there are also similar disagreements on how to diagnose and treat it.[17]

A woman's menstrual cycle is divided into two phases: the follicular phase, which occurs prior to ovulation, and the luteal phase, which begins when the egg is released from the follicle. During the critical luteal phase, the follicle develops into a corpus luteum and releases progesterone, which is necessary to develop the uterine lining. Advocates of LPD believe that in some women the luteal phase is too short to produce enough progesterone to sufficiently develop the endometrium. Their remedy for this seemingly simple problem is to support the body with supplementary progesterone to help the endometrium grow, generally in the form of suppositories or intramuscular injections. Skeptics are, well, skeptical—both that the condition exists at all and that progesterone can help it.

Dozens of studies have sought to answer the question of whether progesterone can prevent miscarriages, and, while a handful of small trials from the 1950s and 1960s have shown some positive effects for women who have experienced three or more miscarriages, the evidence is increasingly falling on the side of the naysayers.[18] Yet puzzlingly, the data has not had a perceptible impact on clinical practice. Despite the fact that a landmark large-scale evaluation of fourteen research studies found *no significant difference* in birth rates between women who received progesterone and those who did not,[19] doctors have continued to prescribe it, and women have continued to ask for it, in hopes that it might help.

The very first, and long overdue, double-blind randomized comprehensive assessment of whether progesterone therapy reduces the risk of miscarriage in women with a history of recurrent miscarriage was finally completed and its findings published in 2016. Known as the PROMISE trial, this groundbreaking international study, the largest clinical trial ever conducted on the subject of recurrent pregnancy loss, involved forty-five clinics treating women ranging in age from eighteen to thirty-nine, all of whom had suffered at least three or more losses. Its major finding can be summed up in one sentence: "[P]rogesterone therapy in the first trimester of pregnancy in women with recurrent miscarriage is of no benefit and, therefore, should not be used in clinical settings."[20]

I suspect that the majority of women who take it have no idea that there is little evidence that progesterone helps maintain a pregnancy. I was prescribed progesterone suppositories with three of my IVF cycles in the United Kingdom and the United States, and (painful) progesterone shots with an additional two. The progesterone shots are so nasty that women lament them daily: "It gets more and more painful each night. It hurts so bad that I literally had tears," commented one woman in the midst of her cycle. "Of all the injections and things that have gone on with this IVF—these progesterone shots are *by far* the worst. I have lumps on both sides and sometimes itch like crazy at the site afterward," remarked another. Women and their partners develop tactics for coping with the difficult shots and readily share successful tips with others: "I used a heating pad for about ten minutes on my rear end before doing the injections. After applying the heat, I'd rub an ice cube inside a sandwich baggie, wrapped in a washcloth, to numb the skin. Then the heating pad went back on my tush afterward to relax the muscle again."

I had naively assumed that my various doctors would not have prescribed progesterone if there was insufficient evidence that it worked, so I never thought to ask. Whether the common practice of prescribing progesterone will continue in the face of this new evidence is yet to be seen.

Progesterone aside, despite years of trial and clinical practice, the evidence is scant that hormonal therapies can help to prevent recurrent miscarriage. Since the risks of many of these timeworn therapies are low, doctors and patients alike continue to turn to them in the absence of alternatives. In addition, when women deliver healthy babies after trying Clomid, letrozole, metformin, or progesterone, they naturally become passionate advocates for the cause. Unfortunately, it is nearly impossible to know with anything approaching certainty whether a specific remedy helped, particularly in light of the fact that even veterans of multiple pregnancy losses have even odds of carrying to term on the next try.

While many women with polycystic ovaries and PCOS go on to carry healthy babies to term, I, unfortunately, was not one of them. Although I did manage to get pregnant several times while on Clomid, I miscarried each and every time. But was the PCOS to blame? As I was to discover, I had several other obstacles in my path, and my once-intense focus on the little string of pearls on my ovaries quickly receded into the background.

Anatomical Factors

I had been trying to have a baby for years before I learned that there are anatomical challenges to both becoming pregnant and carrying to term—and that I, myself, might be facing one. Two of the most common anatomical abnormalities are a misshapen uterus and shortened cervix.

UTERINE ABNORMALITIES

I hated just about everything about my hysterosalpingogram (HSG), a test performed to discover whether all looks right in the uterus and the fallopian tubes are open and in good working order. Although Mr. P had told me the procedure was routine, for some reason I had a bad feeling about it. Richard was traveling on business again, and I had to face it alone, on an unusually gray, even by London standards, sad-looking day. My foreboding increased when I met the doctor who would perform it, which was also inexplicable, as I had subjected myself to poking and prodding for quite some time by then, as well as to uncomfortable examinations (in every sense of the word) by middle-aged, well-pedigreed men and had become quite used to it.

Mr. C, the HSG specialist referred by Mr. P, began the procedure with something called a Cook catheter. He complained to the nurse assisting him about how difficult it was to "cannulate" my cervix, which I later learned meant basically to push the tube through it. I desperately fought to suppress my need to scream as he jabbed me in every possible direction, and I sighed with relief when he finally gave up. My respite was brief, for he came at me with a new tool, which turned out to be a device called a Leech-Wilkinson catheter.

"I suppose you are aware that your uterus is retroverted," he mused.

"No, I wasn't aware," I squeaked. The words I needed to say, the ones that wouldn't leave my head—*What does that mean?*—lay silent.

"Well, it's also T-shaped," he continued. *What?* Silence. He didn't choose to elaborate, and, to this day, I don't know why I didn't ask. I hadn't yet found my voice. He wrapped up the procedure by telling me that my tubes looked fine and that he would send the results to my doctor.

Mr. P shared the report with me at our next appointment. Apparently, Mr. C didn't enjoy the procedure either: "I performed a hysterosalpingogram on this lady for you. It was not particularly easy. She has a difficult cervix to cannulate," his letter began. "Although visualization of the cervix was easy, she has a bell-shaped endocervix with an outlet to the uterine cavity, which was difficult to negotiate with a Cook catheter," he continued. "Accordingly after trying with a tenaculum and probe, failing to insert the Cook catheter I used a Leech-Wilkinson catheter instead. The uterine cavity did not distend very well and it was slightly T-shaped. . . ."

Although neither doctor explained it to me at the time, uterine abnormalities are a known cause of miscarriage. If the uterus is not shaped properly, it may not be receptive to implantation. By injecting dye into the uterus and fallopian tubes, the HSG test indicates the presence of abnormalities that may present obstacles to implantation.

It turned out that my retroverted uterus was not a big deal. Retroverted simply means that the uterus tilts backward instead of forward. One woman among four or five has a retroverted uterus, and it shouldn't cause a problem during pregnancy. A T-shaped uterus, on the other hand, can present real problems. Most commonly seen in women whose mothers took diethylstilbestrol (DES), a synthetic hormone that acts as an endocrine disruptor, to help them conceive, I later learned that the T-shape has a high correlation with failed implantation, miscarriage, and preterm births. Of course, Mr. P didn't mention any of this at the time. Rather, I was told that my uterus was "slightly T-shaped" and nothing to worry about.

A few specialists and tests later, I was asked if I was ever told that I had an arcuate or septate uterus. I proudly responded that I knew I had a retroverted, slightly T-shaped uterus, but no, I had never heard those other words. The HSG test is generally used to diagnose an arcuate or septate uterus, but despite having endured the test, they did not diagnose me at the time.

A typical uterus is often described as being shaped like an upside-down pear, providing a nice big area for a newly fertilized embryo to implant. An arcuate uterus has a slight dip at the top, rendering a less elegant, but apparently only marginally less welcoming home for the burrowing embryo. Many women with arcuate uteruses have kids without much trouble. In the case of a septate uterus, however, the dip reaches down farther, starting to form a wall between the two halves of the uterus and impeding the blood flow that is necessary for implantation. Women with septate uteruses have a lot of difficulty having kids. Many doctors advocate treating a septate uterus with surgery (a procedure called hysteroscopic metroplasty or just metroplasty) to remove the offending tissue forming the wall. While believed to be highly effective, this surgery is not without controversy, both due to risk and a lack of double-blind randomized trials proving its efficacy.

Frustratingly, in certain women, it is hard to tell the difference. Apparently, I was one of those. In my case, I was advised that my oddly shaped uterus was likely arcuate and therefore not a problem, and that I should move on.

When I first met Anna, the social worker who counsels teens, she visibly shuddered when she mentioned her HSG test.

"Wasn't it awful?" I asked.

"Well, I had three," she replied, "and three surgeries. Beyond awful."

Anna's first HSG test revealed a suspected septum in the uterus, which she was advised to have removed before she tried to conceive. She complied, and was eager to start trying for a baby as soon as possible after the procedure. Her doctor insisted that she have a second HSG test to make sure she was ready; the test revealed lots of scar tissue, yet it did not appear that the surgeon had removed the septum. Anna had a second surgery, which she was told was successful. She then hopped on the fertility roller coaster. Nearly two years later, a new fertility specialist insisted she have another HSG test, which revealed a remaining septum that was three centimeters long. Anna went back under the knife a third time. Her septum finally vanquished, she began her IVF cycle as soon as possible after the surgery, and gave birth to a beautiful, healthy baby almost thirty-six weeks later.

In Anna's case, identifying and fixing the septate uterus were likely key to her success.

CERVICAL INCOMPETENCE

Cervical incompetence, also known as cervical insufficiency, is the second major anatomical disorder routinely treated in an effort to prevent miscarriage. The cervix is the lower part of the uterus that opens to the vagina. Normally closed, as a pregnancy progresses, the cervix gradually softens and opens in preparation for birth. An "incompetent" cervix is one that shortens too much or opens too soon, making it difficult for the uterus to hold the baby inside. In the worst-case scenario, the baby is born far too early, before it is capable of life outside the womb.

For nearly fifty years, doctors have treated cervical incompetence by inserting a cerclage, or surgical stitch, to literally close the door to the outside world and keep the baby inside, provided that the mother is early enough in her pregnancy—generally up to sixteen weeks, but in certain emergency cases up to the twenty-fourth week.[21] It is considered too risky to perform later on in the pregnancy, and many women who are found to have shortened cervixes in their second and third trimesters find themselves instead confined to bed rest, itself not without complications, including loss of muscle strength, joint pain, and depression.

As with so many areas surrounding infertility and miscarriage, there is no consensus on why cervical incompetence occurs, and also no agreement on whether cerclage works. There is, however, agreement on this procedure's risks, which include infection, vaginal bleeding, a tear in the cervix, premature labor and birth, and miscarriage.

Also in common with many other aspects of infertility and miscarriage, the verdict on success rates is inconclusive, with a few small studies indicating a benefit in the case of urgent cerclage (performed upon diagnosis of a shortened cervix)[22] and numerous other studies concluding that there is no benefit to either elective (chosen because of past losses, as opposed to demonstrated physical need, and usually inserted at twelve to fourteen weeks) or urgent cerclage.[23] There is no data at all on the efficacy of emergency cerclage. Performed in the event of a feared preterm labor when the cervix dilates early, emergency cerclage is, by its very nature, performed only in crises, rendering controlled studies virtually impossible.

The success of cerclage has also been found to vary based on whether the mother is carrying one or multiple babies. Women carrying a singleton with a shortened cervix and previous preterm birth had a greater chance of making it to term and a much lower chance of miscarriage when they received a cerclage.[24] But there is no evidence of similar success for women carrying multiples. To the contrary, whether the women in question actually had a shortened cervix or were just at risk by virtue of carrying multiples, five clinical trials found no improvement in preventing preterm births or deaths.[25]

Yvette's story is heartbreaking. At age thirty-two, after two years of unsuccessfully trying to have a baby, she and her husband, Karl, both Catholic, went to a renowned fertility clinic for an initial consultation. Not quite ready for intervention, they opted to first try herbs, acupuncture, and dietary changes. Yvette felt great and loved her treatments, but another year rolled by and she still was not pregnant. After considerable discussion and struggle, they eventually made the decision to move on to IVF. Concerned about the risk of multiples, her doctors transferred only two embryos to Yvette, despite having the luxury of twenty-one embryos available to them. Concerned that her blood tests revealed high HCG (the earliest indicator of both a healthy pregnancy and of multiples), Yvette and Karl awaited their first ultrasound, anxious that they might learn they were having twins. At their eight-week scan, they were startled to see not two heartbeats, as they feared, but three. One of the embryos had split, and Yvette was pregnant with triplets. At her eighteen-week checkup, she discovered that her cervix was shortening, and the doctor recommended a cerclage and bed rest.

Optimistic that the cerclage would keep her babies safe, at least for the next few weeks, Yvette committed to bed rest. At week twenty, her cervix was still shrinking and Yvette was having contractions. Her high-risk neonatal specialist wanted her to make it at least to week twenty-one, which, with cervix stretched to the stitch, she miraculously did. Yet in the face of all their best efforts—which in addition to cerclage also included intravenous cocktails of magnesium, Celebrex, terbutaline and Procardia—to keep the babies inside, just three days after hitting the week-twenty-one milestone, Yvette gave birth to their three precious angels, who tragically left them the same day.

Antiphospholipid Syndrome

The blood clots that led Mr. Raj Rai to diagnose me with antiphospholipid syndrome (APS) at the Recurrent Miscarriage Clinic are believed to lead to miscarriages, premature delivery, and stillbirths, although the linkage is not yet well understood. The first commonly accepted explanation of the relationship between APS and miscarriage is that the clots, which are small enough to cross the placenta (which provides vital nutrients to the fetus), essentially starve the fetus and deprive it of vital oxygen. The second major theory holds that the hallmark antibodies may prevent the fetus from implanting properly in the womb in the first place. In either event, the correlation to pregnancy loss seems crystal clear.

Fortunately, APS is the most significant cause of recurrent miscarriage that can be successfully remedied, which is a relief to women such as myself who are diagnosed with it. APS is the primary cause of at least 15 percent (and some believe as high as 50 percent) of recurrent miscarriages. With proper diagnosis and treatment, the pregnancy-loss rate among women with APS has fallen from 80 percent in the 1980s to only 20 to 30 percent today, an absolute miracle for many women.[26]

In a study of women with APS who had at least three or more consecutive losses, it was discovered that *90 percent would miscarry again without treatment.*[27] The researchers established that women taking low-dose aspirin together with low-molecular-weight heparin were far more likely to have a baby (71 percent success rate) than those taking aspirin alone (42 percent success rate).[28] The results were astonishing and hailed as a breakthrough worth celebrating.

Unlike baby aspirin, which is easily swallowed daily, heparin (most commonly known by the brand names Clexane and Lovenox) must be injected subcutaneously twice a day. Definitely not ideal for a needle-phobe like me, but as with acupuncture and IVF, when I want something badly enough, I get my head around it. I learned to inject myself with Clexane and even became adept at finding creative new spots to puncture myself as my once-pristine white tummy, which had rarely seen the light of day, turned purple, blue, and charcoal gray as the bruises layered upon one another.

Additionally, in 2017, news broke about the first new drug to improve pregnancy rates in women with APS since the advent of aspirin and heparin. Though at an early stage of development, a small-scale study in London found that pravastatin, a medicine intended to lower cholesterol that has been used for almost thirty years to prevent cardiovascular disease, looks extremely promising in assisting women with APS to have healthy babies.[29]

Other Immunological Problems

First, I had been diagnosed with polycystic ovaries, and Clomid was supposed to be my answer. After that, I learned about my irregular uterus, but it was deemed to be arcuate, and therefore not a serious problem. My *real* trouble, we were next told, was the antiphospholipid syndrome. But that wouldn't hold us back; I simply needed aspirin and heparin to solve that one. Yet none of the treatments seemed to make a difference. I still couldn't manage to hang on to a single pregnancy. So by the time I first heard of natural killer cells, after four miscarriages, I was more than willing to believe that taming my rogue killer cells held the answer.

According to the controversial theory of natural killer cells, an overactive immune system detects a newly formed fetus as a foreign and unwelcome intrusion and essentially attacks and destroys the invader. The treatment for this problem involves intravenous infusion of immunoglobulin, known as IVIG, which suppresses the immune system, some believe dangerously.

I was blissfully unaware at the time that in a field riddled with contradictory studies and flagrant disagreements, the debates surrounding the role of natural killer cells—whether they cause miscarriage at all, let alone whether certain remedies are effective—steal the controversy crown. While there is general agreement on the impact of APS, itself an autoimmune problem, on pregnancy, the consensus on the role of immunology in miscarriage stops there. For more than fifty years, passionate supporters and equally ardent detractors have clashed over both the question of whether a mother's immune system may view her fledgling fetus as a trespasser and attack it, and if so, whether immunotherapy treatments could prevent such attacks. The conflict makes this one of the most challenging medical topics for aspiring parents to get their heads around.

Reproductive immunology treatment, while growing in leaps and bounds, is offered in a relatively cloistered world consisting largely of specialized clinics staffed by doctors engaged in cutting-edge practice. Entering this world feels a little bit like being welcomed into a secret club. With well-respected clinics stating that immune mechanisms account for 50 percent of miscarriage and claiming a success rate of 80 percent in treating these problems,[30] it is very hard to disregard the potential. On top of the success rates, the rationale is alluring and easy to understand: rogue natural killer, or NK, cells inhabiting the mother's uterus attack the fetus, treating it as a foreign body. The treatment centers around the theory that these overly aggressive natural killer cells can be tamed, creating a hospitable environment for the fetus.

The problem is that consistent scientific studies to back up the theory are conspicuously absent. Since the earliest forays into framing and treating the alleged immunology problem, treatments have been offered to women without sufficient evidence that they either worked or, at a minimum, would do no harm. Lymphocyte immune therapy (LIT), the first widespread treatment protocol for miscarriage deemed to be caused by the immune system, was ultimately, after decades of use, banned by the FDA. Initially considered a major theoretical breakthrough in the world of understanding miscarriage, the idea behind LIT is relatively appealing to the layperson: a woman's immune system reacts hostilely to the baby in her womb because it contains the genes of the father, foreign to her body; injecting the mother with the father's white blood cells will make her more accepting of the foreigner. After years of testing on mice, rats, and hamsters, the first human baby conceived following LIT was born in 1980. Under the care of Dr. Alan Beer—considered the father of reproductive immunology in the United States—the baby's mother, who was thirty-nine and had experienced seven miscarriages, received an infusion of her husband's blood cells, and at age forty gave birth to their healthy son.

At the same time, across the pond, James Mowbray, a researcher at St. Mary's Hospital in London, organized the first placebo-controlled, double-blind trial of LIT. The small trial, which assessed forty-seven women, divided them randomly into two groups, one of which received lymphocytes (white blood cells) from their husbands, the other of which received their own. Promisingly, 78 percent of women in the treatment group had a live birth, compared to 37 percent in the placebo group.[31]

All looked fantastically bright for the future of LIT. Dr. Beer and his reproductive immunology treatments rose in fame as more "Beer babies" were born. *People* magazine ran a cover story about him called "Injection of Hope," while national TV networks devoted airtime to his new methods.[32] Clinics around the nation and the world began to offer LIT, and an article in *Newsweek* called the progress in preventing miscarriage "little short of spectacular."[33]

But somewhat ironically, at almost the same time, a study emerged from Norway on a treatment protocol that had even more favorable results than LIT, with 86 percent of women in the treatment group carrying to term, compared to only 33 percent in the control group, among a population that had previously experienced three consecutive miscarriages.[34] The variable in the Norwegian study: tender loving care. It turned out that weekly visits to check the mothers' and babies' vitals provided assurance that the pregnancies were progressing smoothly. This "optimal psychological support" presumably reduced stress and anxiety, and proved as successful as the invasive LIT intervention. Seven years later, a team at a recurrent miscarriage clinic in Auckland, New Zealand, conducted a similar study, providing "formal supportive care" to their treatment group and routine care to a control group through the patients' first trimesters. Startlingly, among a population of women who averaged four previous miscarriages, the Auckland team found the exact same result: 86 percent of the treatment group carried to term, versus 33 percent of the control group.[35]

The Norwegian "tender loving care" study, together with growing concerns about the risks inherent in blood transfusions—such as transferring an undetected infection or triggering an immune rejection reaction—and a lack of clear-cut evidence that LIT worked, prompted the organization of a large-scale, four-year study, known as the Recurrent Miscarriage Study, or REMIS, intended to shed definitive light on the effectiveness of the therapy. The results were much anticipated, but the trial was never completed. Quite unusually, the US government terminated the study when the reviewers noted that, contrary to what the researchers and public expected, the control group had significantly better results than the treatment group.[36] On January 30, 2002, the FDA sent a letter to clinics administering LIT instructing them to refrain from any administration of LIT unless given in connection with approved clinical investigations, citing concern that the treatment may produce a *higher* rate of miscarriage and that it presented risks to the recipient.[37]

Despite the scientific evidence to the contrary, doctors and patients alike, led by Dr. Beer, were undeterred in their belief that immunology might hold the key to preventing miscarriage, and efforts to crack the code continued in earnest. Following the same theory of taming a woman's immune system by essentially diluting it with cells from another, doctors turned toward a protocol that was already approved by the FDA, albeit for a different purpose. Instead of their husbands' white cells, this entailed infusing women with antibodies pooled from several people through IVIG.

Notwithstanding the absence of proof that it works, IVIG remains today the frontline treatment for miscarriages believed to be caused by natural killer cells. Opponents of the practice point out numerous flaws on the pathway to supporting IVIG for preventing pregnancy loss. First, challengers note that while there is no disagreement surrounding the existence of uterine natural killer cells, the function of these uterine NK cells is completely unknown, and a link between the cells and miscarriage has not been conclusively demonstrated. On top of that, because natural killer cells found in the uterus are different from NK cells found in blood, critics argue that measuring the amount of NK cells in blood will not shed light on what is happening in the uterus. Some of the world's leading miscarriage experts note that measuring the number of uterine NK cells through the blood tests currently in use "is akin to estimating the number and activity of black cabs in Trafalgar Square by analysing red minicabs circulating on the M25."[38]* And finally, and perhaps most persuasively, experts emphasize that there is no evidence to show that immunological suppression treatments such as IVIG and steroids, which present known risks to both mother and baby, are successful. In fact, a Cochrane review of twenty randomized controlled trials in eleven countries found that *none* of the immunotherapy treatments provided a significant benefit in improving live birth rates or lowering the risk of future miscarriage among women who have recurrent miscarriages.[39] Neither the American Society of Reproductive Medicine nor the British Royal College of Obstetricians and Gynaecologists supports its use.

---

*Or for Americans, akin to estimating the number of people in Times Square by the number of cars on the Long Island Expressway.

Yet proponents of immunotherapy are not dissuaded. Citing their personal success stories and often their own clinics' statistics regarding successful pregnancies following treatment, many doctors advocating IVIG maintain that they are ahead of the curve in understanding a mechanism that plays a clear and significant role in miscarriage. "In my opinion, it is very regrettable and unfortunate that so many patients are denied the ability to go from 'infertility to family' simply because (for whatever reason) so many reproductive specialists refuse to address the role of immunologic factors in the genesis of intractable reproductive dysfunction," Dr. Geoffrey Sher, a renowned fertility expert, says on his website. "Hopefully this will change . . . and the sooner the better."[40] Some clinics go much further, claiming that "Intravenous immunoglobulin (IVIG) has been established as one of the most effective treatments for multiple miscarriage. . . . A large percentage of women who have experienced recurrent miscarriage have found that IVIG is an effective solution to the immunologic causes of miscarriage."[41]

In 2005, I found myself seduced by the promise of IVIG. After all my discoveries and failures, I believed that I had found the missing piece. What else did I have to hold on to? Dr. Beer argued that women with recurrent miscarriages caused by immunological factors effectively "become serial killers of their own babies."[42] If there was even a slight chance that what he said was true, how could I not try to fight that?

Sarah and Evan are grateful for the reproductive immunology treatments. After three miscarriages, all following natural conceptions, they decided to see a fertility specialist, who informed them that Sarah had a blood-clotting disorder. Her doctor prescribed the blood thinner Lovenox to be started immediately, before conception. Sarah became pregnant a fourth time and continued the Lovenox, but it failed to prevent her fourth miscarriage. This devastating loss prompted them to leave their comfortable Boston clinic and excellent Massachusetts insurance plan and head to a famous reproductive immunology clinic in New York City, where they had their "first glimpse of fertility as a business." While their Massachusetts insurance had covered $150,000 of Sarah's treatment costs in Boston, their consultation in NY, together with two phone calls and lab tests, cost $6,000 (paid out of pocket), despite the fact that their doctor ate lunch through their meeting and called Sarah the wrong name. But it may have been worth it. Sarah was advised to do an IVF cycle while taking Lovenox (daily) to thin her blood, steroids (daily) while also undergoing IVIG (every three weeks) to tame her immune system, and preimplantation genetic testing (PGS) to select a healthy embryo. In the end, they had one healthy, chromosomally normal embryo transferred into Sarah's immune-suppressed womb, and welcomed their baby eight months later.

Sarah and Evan will never know if it was the immunotherapy that gave them their baby. Perhaps it was the genetic testing, which helped in selecting a normal embryo. Or maybe it was luck.

One of the greatest obstacles to evaluating miscarriage therapies is the fact that many, if not the majority, of women who conceive will carry to term with no intervention, even if they have miscarried in the past. In fact, studies indicate that 95 percent of women who miscarry will conceive again in the two years following the miscarriage, and that approximately 85 percent of women who have experienced one miscarriage and as many as 70 percent of women with recurrent pregnancy loss will succeed in subsequent pregnancies.[43] Ironically, in much the same way that most miscarriages still go unexplained, pregnancy success following recurrent miscarriage can also go unexplained. This conundrum highlights the need for large-scale, randomized double-blind studies to test the effectiveness of treatments. But only a few such studies have been conducted, and patients are rarely made aware of their findings. Rather, doctors tend to measure the efficacy of a treatment against their own patient pool, or against an individual patient's own history, which may or may not have validity for others.

There are untold variables to every pregnancy, and patients also tend to use their own success as a yardstick against which to measure practices. If a woman carries to term after taking aspirin and heparin every day, or has a baby following surgery to fix a septate uterus, or after enduring IVIG infusions, she will ascribe her success to the relevant treatment. But if a doctor tells a pregnant woman to drink orange juice every day throughout her pregnancy and she carries to term, does that mean that the orange juice prevented miscarriage?

Compounding these "rational" problems is the ever-present reality that dealing with repeated losses of desperately longed-for babies does not place most people in a rational or analytical mind-set. With each miscarriage, I felt more and more distressed, but also more determined, and increasingly open to trying drastic measures. I would try anything and everything. With any sliver of hope of success, I was willing to throw a Hail Mary. Doing nothing never felt like an option to me.

Yet ironically, the hard-learned lessons from treatments such as DES and LIT teach us that opting to do nothing—which can be much harder than trying something, anything—is often the wiser choice.

It takes three to make a child.

e. e. cummings

Down the Rabbit Hole of
Third-Party Parenting

Gestational Surrogacy

*W*hen my mother first suggested I consider using a surrogate, I absolutely was not ready to hear it, despite four miscarriages and many known pregnancy obstacles. This was before anyone ever really talked about surrogacy—before Nicole Kidman and Sarah Jessica Parker, before *Baby Mama* hit the big screen. She mentioned it gingerly on the phone, telling me how excited their good friends were that their son and his male partner had just had a baby with a surrogate mother; she e-mailed me articles from the *New York Times,* her equivalent of the Bible. I ignored her, in that very special way that daughters do with mothers. But my mother had succeeded; the seed had been planted.

After the fifth miscarriage, Richard decided to step in as well. We had long talked about the possibility of adoption, and with five miscarriages and five years under our belt, and IVF clearly failing us, he tenderly told me it was time to explore this path. I wanted to be comfortable with it, but the truth was I was just not ready to give up on biological children. I had been pregnant five times! I *knew* I could have a baby. Looking back, I think that after the heartbreak of grieving over five miscarriages, I had the strange but fixed notion that a successful natural-born child would somehow wipe out the pain of the five I had lost. In a way, I felt I was fighting for the life of the same baby each time. I know this is irrational, but it is how I felt.

In this respect too we were not alone, although we did not know it then. Married nine years, after four IVF cycles and four miscarriages, Paula's husband, Derrick, was ready to give up on the fertility industry. Facing too much heartbreak, too many expenses, and too little assurance of a baby to take home, like Richard, he was ready, and eager, to pursue adoption. But Paula wasn't there yet. The fiery and determined Brazilian-Italian told me: "You'd have had to kill me then for me to give up on having my own child." Although theoretically open to considering adoption in the future, like me, she was too focused on trying to get her body to conceive to give any other path a chance.

Living in an international city like London, I frequently heard reports of triumphant successes in countries that were not too far away, and I felt that, having come this far, we owed it to ourselves to explore clinics overseas. Although not ready to admit it, I also had my mother's voice in the back of my head. . . .

Richard, a consummate option maximizer, convinced me that we should pursue all the options simultaneously. We began the process to get approved to adopt in the United Kingdom, starting with required adoption classes and a home study with a social worker, a process that takes on average nine months to complete in the United Kingdom as opposed to one to three months in the United States. We also started exploring avenues to finding a baby to adopt, a search that can take years. We quickly settled on Russia as our preferred country, in part because we are both of Eastern European descent, and largely because we had connections from our professional lives to people who were well positioned to help us expedite the process there. We had each been working on projects in Moscow on and off for a number of years, and by 2005, we were spending nearly half of our time there.

Ironically, although we complained bitterly about Britain's required group adoption classes at the start—primarily about waking up early on invariably gray Saturday mornings and taking the Tube to South London to spend the better part of our precious free day in the comparably gray concrete classroom building—we came to appreciate the importance of urging onto prospective adopters the responsibilities and unique challenges many adoptive parents face.

At the same time, in contravention of the adoption rules (which required that potential adoptive parents stop all other efforts to have a child), I researched fertility clinics in Spain, Cyprus, and the United States and started to tiptoe into the complicated world of surrogacy, a realm in which regulation and practice vary from country to country and clinic to clinic, and strangers are involved in your most intimate affairs. In addition to the already time-consuming task of evaluating the performance of the clinics, I compared the medical regimes, legal ramifications, costs, and practical aspects of how to find a surrogate in the United States and the United Kingdom, the two countries that were home to me.

Since Richard and I were living in London, we ultimately decided to pursue surrogacy in the United Kingdom so that we could fully participate in the pregnancy, see the little heartbeat on the ultrasound scan, follow the milestones. But the United Kingdom had its own complications. Our doctor at the Lister refused to perform gestational surrogacy, saying that it would not be approved by the hospital's ethics committee. Of course, that same clinic *paid* healthy young women to "donate" their own eggs and allowed would-be parents to *buy* eggs— transactions that last a lifetime—with no ethical concerns; but they had a problem allowing a woman to voluntarily carry an embryo made up of *my* egg and *my husband's* sperm and then give *our* baby back to us? A favor, albeit a huge one, that lasts nine months? We were told that in contrast to the almost universal (apart from the very religious) acceptance of egg and sperm donation, controversy persisted regarding the question of whether a woman should be allowed to "rent" her womb, a practice critics have accused of being akin to selling babies. This response was particularly frustrating in light of the fact that surrogates in the United Kingdom, by law, are not permitted to be paid.

Once again, it was time to find a new clinic and a new doctor.

Dr. Joel Batzofin, a South African–born, New York–based fertility specialist, opened our trans-Atlantic phone conversation with "Your buns are fine, but your oven is broken." He later asked, "Do you want to carry your baby or be a mother to your baby?" Aside from his stellar credentials—after university in South Africa, he was educated at Harvard Medical School and Baylor College of Medicine, followed by a stint on the faculty at Stanford University—and twenty-odd years of experience leading top fertility clinics, his warmth and compassion won me over. By the end of our conversation, I had a new doctor and a new plan. It was nearing Thanksgiving 2005. I intended to go to New York to see him just after the New Year.

The visit didn't happen as planned. By December, I was pregnant again—having naturally conceived.

How much had changed since that Thanksgiving in New York with my parents in 2000. Now, five years later, the United States was involved in two wars, and I was waging an ongoing battle to have a baby. In 2000, I'd spent New Year's Eve hoping the year would find me pregnant, and now I spent my New Year's Eve worried that I was losing time by *being* pregnant. I wanted to be joyous, but with my track record, anxiety ruled the day; if I miscarried again, it would only prolong the wait before I could try with this promising new doctor in New York supervising my care.

As it turned out, I didn't have to wait too long. Just one week into 2006, I had my sixth miscarriage.

It might be hard to imagine that one could greet a miscarriage with relief, but I did. Strangely, I knew that this miscarriage would be my route to actually having a child. Carrying no longer seemed important. I wanted to be a mother to my child.

The adoption and surrogacy alternatives suddenly took on new meaning for me. I devoured agency websites, online communities and blogs, scouring the Internet and bookstores for any and all information. I became addicted to www.intendedparents.com and www.surromomsonline.com, matching sites for surrogates and intended parents. I was a lurker. I read profiles. I read stories. I checked Intended Parents regularly, but there were no surrogates registered in the United Kingdom.

While finding a surrogate in the United States was easier than in the United Kingdom, working with a surrogate in the States seemed complicated, expensive, and legally dicey, as the rules varied drastically from state to state, and it was not assured in many jurisdictions that I would be legally recognized as the mother.

Given all the medical challenges, legal obstacles, and often complex administrative needs, few couples or individuals choose to proceed on their own. There are, in 2017, more than four hundred agencies in the United States alone offering egg donation, sperm donation, or surrogacy services, and there are law firms as well that specialize in surrogacy contracts. Agencies can help with every aspect of the process, from selecting a donor to managing communications with a surrogate. For many, the support that a good agency provides is invaluable, especially when dealing with a surrogate at a distance.

When we began to seriously consider surrogacy in 2006, at Dr. Batzofin's suggestion, I spoke to Melissa Brisman, a nationally recognized reproductive law specialist, who helped me understand the landscape. I studied agency websites. I learned of the need for a clear and detailed contract covering every aspect of the relationship, and every imaginable and unimaginable eventuality: compensation, reimbursable expenses, number of embryos to be transferred, guidelines for selective reduction or termination if necessary, extra compensation in the event of twins, reduced compensation for a miscarriage, travel restrictions, dietary rules, and in some cases even how much caffeine a surrogate is allowed to consume.

I felt an overwhelming need to control the process as much as possible, handling everything myself, without an agency, in no small part because the agencies seemed inexplicably expensive to me. The issues at times were overwhelming: lawyers, contracts, distance, travel costs, and most important, potential custody issues. Pursuing a US surrogate was not only daunting in terms of time, money, and complexity, it was far away. It was hard enough to contemplate someone else carrying my baby; it was simply a step too far to imagine that I wouldn't be there, wouldn't participate, wouldn't see the thrilling ultrasound scans and feel the baby kick.

Faced with the dilemma of a doctor we were excited about in the United States and our desire for a local (although yet unidentified) surrogate, Richard and I invented our own solution: an American clinic and a British surrogate.

Unlike in the United States, where surrogacy is a profitable commercial enterprise, it was, and still is, illegal to pay or advertise for surrogates in the United Kingdom, making it far more difficult to find them, as I had learned through my fruitless efforts. Paying third-party agencies is also prohibited, further frustrating the process. Fortuitously, near the beginning of our search, the BBC ran a show on surrogacy, examining the different laws and procedures in the United States and United Kingdom. The show specifically mentioned Intended Parents, the website that I had perused for countless hours. By a stroke of magnificent luck, some bighearted potential English surrogates must have stayed home that night, watching the telly, for four new English surrogates signed onto the site the next day. Thrilled, I wrote to three of them immediately and spoke to each on the phone. I had a clear favorite. Catherine had one child, who was the light of her life, and had seriously contemplated surrogacy before. Moved by the obvious need in Britain, she was thinking about helping a family. Just a few weeks after I contacted her, Richard and I met Catherine in a pub around the corner from our house. Could this be the woman who would carry our baby?

Catherine was petite with short brown hair. She was shaking as we met at the pub, every bit as nervous as we were. We talked about the weather (rain), the north of England (gray), and her love of gardening, particularly flowers. We learned that she was the single mother of a ten-year old daughter, and that she had trained as a chef. She worked at a large department store and dreamed of opening her own flower shop or café. We tiptoed around the elephant in the room. We liked her—a lot. We hoped she liked us.

Fortunately, she did.

Many conversations later, with the very helpful assistance of a non-profit (as legally required) group called COTS (Childlessness Overcome Through Surrogacy), it was official. We were really going to do this. Now somewhat expert in surrogacy law, I drafted our own contracts, spelling out the process: Starting in England with hormone treatments, we would all travel to New York for the egg harvest (Dr. Batzofin collects the healthy eggs from me), fertilization (egg meets sperm in petri dish), and embryo transfer (Dr. Batzofin puts the best embryos in Catherine five days later). We would compensate Catherine for her expenses and loss of earnings, but under the law, could not otherwise pay her. As for custody, we would apply for a parental order acknowledging me as the mother, and enabling me to be named as mother on the birth certificate along with Richard as father.

There were complications, to be sure—emotional this time, rather than physical. Catherine panicked. Her daughter panicked. I panicked. All at different times of course. The clinic called me in London near the end of my medication cycle—meaning I was fully loaded with hormones to develop as many eggs as possible—to warn me that they were concerned that she might not go through with it. Yet many e-mails, phone calls, meetings, tears, and days later, Richard, Catherine, and I all got on the plane bound for New York and Dr. Batzofin. We told a few people, but not too many. It all seemed so . . . experimental.

I had another "great" IVF cycle, although it would be a lie to say it wasn't completely nerve-racking. There were unexpected decisions to be made. My uterine lining, which had been inadequately thin for many cycles and was one of the key indicators for my needing a surrogate, was "sufficient" this time, and the doctor raised the question of my trying again. Should I attempt carrying myself? Should we both carry? If we transferred two embryos to each of us that could result in potentially four babies! It might also lead our surrogate to opt out. And could I bear another miscarriage? No, we decided. We would stick to the plan.

We all stayed at my parents' house on Long Island, where every afternoon, we would anxiously wait for a critical phone call from the clinic. First, it was the condition of the eggs. Then, the number that fertilized. After that, the quality of the growing embryos. Each call was more terrifying than the last. And finally, the PGS results.

Again, the numbers dwindled at an alarming rate:

Twenty-eight eggs retrieved
Seventeen fertilized
Thirteen mature enough to be tested
Three chromosomally normal

With each diminishing number, we were overwhelmed by our new understanding of how low our chances really were, and how much time we had been wasting the past few years without this critical information. Of the twenty-eight eggs retrieved, only *three* were normal, an unusually low number—and they were not the embryos that looked the best, by a long shot. Two girls and one boy. Given our history of failures, I wanted to transfer them all. Dr. Batzofin strongly counseled against it.

With a good carrier (not me), there was no reason they shouldn't stick. He urged us to transfer the two best-quality embryos to Catherine. I agonized all night.

I needn't have bothered. By the time we got to the clinic the next day, the male embryo had arrested. Before I processed what was happening, Dr. Batzofin transferred two embryos into Catherine's practically perfect womb (a phrase that stuck when Mr. Braithwaite first joked with her in London). He was extremely confident. One of them, he told us, was a "super embryo."

Two weeks later, his confidence was confirmed. At last we had a viable pregnancy without my many medical issues getting in the way. And what a difference it made.

As I knew it was extremely difficult for some women, I was worried about how I might react to a surrogate carrying our child instead of me. But in our case, as with many others I met, it was not only never a problem, it was pure joy. When we went to the ultrasound scans back in London, we were excited rather than nervous. Each checkup brought good news, not the bleak announcements to which we had become accustomed. When Mr. Braithwaite smilingly told Catherine that everything looked perfect, she replied, "I bet you say that to everyone." We were quick to assure her that definitely was not the case! Friends and family worried that a surrogate might become attached to the baby she was carrying. Yet as the months passed and Catherine and we grew closer, never for a single moment did any one of us confuse whose baby it was.

On December 30, 2006, nearly three weeks ahead of schedule, Catherine went into labor. Richard and I rushed to Ormskirk and District General Hospital near her hometown of Southport to join her. Several hours later, we welcomed into our world our beautiful, perfect, healthy, and so longed-for daughter, Alexandra.

A surrogate birth is magical, and rather than feeling like it was "second best," we felt unbelievably privileged to be part of such an extraordinary experience. We participated in every moment of the amazing arrival of our long-awaited baby, along with our wonderful new extended English family. Catherine's mother—who helpfully was a midwife—daughter, and sisters showered us with love and welcomed us into their homes as their own family. Our hospital experience was phenomenal, and although unorthodox, felt entirely normal to us. We stood by Catherine's side in the delivery room, sometimes holding her hand, sometimes giving her space. Richard cut the umbilical cord as I gazed on in wonder. Catherine and I shared a double maternity room, and while I had baby Alexandra by my side and received all the support and copious advice a new mother would normally receive in Britain, Catherine received the tender care that a woman who has just delivered deserves. I learned to breastfeed (I had taken essential hormones to make this possible), and Richard and I together were taught to bathe and swaddle our new baby, and to make a proper bottle.

After years of failed bets, Richard and I had finally hit the trifecta: with Catherine and her amazing family, a smooth delivery, and caregivers who were kind beyond imagination, we knew we were the lucky ones. We left the hospital on New Year's Day 2007, Richard looking a bit worse for wear after ringing in the New Year with Catherine's party-loving, gambling grandmother, and we headed to our London home amazed at our good fortune. The next few weeks and months were busy with the normal newborn-baby things, as well as a few extras—registering her birth in the United Kingdom, applying for a British passport, establishing maternity in the United Kingdom through a parental order (all surprisingly easy, especially with the help of a knowledgeable colleague and friend), trying to get US citizenship for our baby (unexpectedly difficult, despite our both being US citizens).

When Alexandra was a few months old, Catherine called one day to talk about Number Two. *Number Two?* She knew we wanted to have two children, she said, and she'd rather do it sooner than later. The idea of having another baby before Alexandra was even eighteen months old was terrifying, but the thought of losing Catherine was even more daunting. We decided to go again in November and stay in New York through Thanksgiving. By this time, Catherine had a boyfriend, Paul, and he joined us as well. It was quite cozy, all of us together in my parents' two-bedroom apartment.

We thought the second time would be easier than the first. Same doctor, same drug protocols, same surrogate. Unfortunately, it didn't work that way. Our IVF cycle yielded only eight eggs, five of which fertilized and developed into embryos. I picked away at my nails waiting for the PGS results. Zero normal. None. No transfer. I was only a year and a half older than I had been the year before. How could we have *no* normal embryos?

After discussion with Dr. Batzofin and his embryologist, we decided that the frozen embryos we had from our second (free) try with Mr. P offered our best chance of success. They were frozen in 2004, when I was four years younger. We believed they should have a higher chance of being normal.

In yet another foray into unknown territory, I dove into the complex world of transferring embryos across international borders in a portable high-tech freezer. Luckily, I found Krystos, my Greek shipping savior. It turns out that transporting embryos is almost as difficult as producing them. While Krystos amazed me with his ability to surmount nearly every obstacle—and there were many—there was one even he couldn't surmount: Catherine called. She was out as a surrogate. She was going to marry Paul. Although he was very supportive and proud of her having helped us to have Alexandra, he could not deal with his new bride being pregnant with someone else's baby. It was hard to argue with that. Now what?

Once again, my type A personality kicked into high gear. I was on the surrogate sites every night. Like in the world of online dating, demand was growing, and by early 2008, it was becoming much more competitive to find a surrogate match in England, especially one willing to travel to the United States for treatment. We opened ourselves to the

US option. Eventually, I found a wonderful potential surrogate named Brenda. She was from Pennsylvania, which I knew was a surrogacy favorable state, married (also surrogacy favorable), and had already been a successful surrogate (perfect). We struck up a friendly e-mail relationship and spoke on the phone. It was decided that we would meet in New York and try with the frozen embryos. Brenda was sure it would work; she never failed to get pregnant before. But she had never met my embryos.

The lab thawed our embryos, and we were planning for a day five transfer, after the results of the all-important genetic testing were available. Bad news again. The embryos were all useless, albeit in different ways. Some were frozen improperly (no surprise, given our experience with that incompetent first clinic), and some had complex chromosomal abnormalities. We looked at the slides with the doctor and embryologist. Even to the untrained eye, it was clear. It was a disaster.

Undaunted, Brenda agreed to try one more time. We scheduled what Richard and I agreed would be our *last IVF cycle ever*, for the summer of 2008. We spent the month of July in New York doing another fresh cycle, this time with the drug protocol boosted higher than ever before (as is common in repeat IVF cyclers), in an attempt to produce more eggs. We were looking for the proverbial needle in the haystack, and we needed to search through lots of hay. Other than feeling like hell, which is an understatement, the cycle went well. We had eight eggs and eight embryos.

But, once again, none were normal. Not one. Zero.

It was time to give up, Dr. Batzofin said. The embryologist echoed his opinion. My consultants in London echoed his opinion. My obstetrician and gynecologist friends at Brigham and Women's in Boston echoed his opinion. I had no more good eggs. It was hard news to swallow. But we reluctantly decided that we had reached the end of the road. And we felt lucky every single day to have Alexandra.

Surrogacy

Ever since Phoebe, pregnant with her brother's triplets, burst into American homes in season four of the ever-popular *Friends,* third-party parenting—comprising egg donation, sperm donation, traditional surrogates (the surrogate carries her own egg) and gestational surrogates (the surrogate carries the egg of the intended mother or a donor)—has caught the imagination of Hollywood and infiltrated mainstream media. Unfortunately, lawmakers, medical administrators, and policy makers remain many steps behind, with regulation of third-party parenting varying widely not only from country to country, but also, within the unregulated United States, from state to state. In some states, for instance, the birth mother of a surrogate baby is recognized as the mother of the baby, regardless of intent or biology, and the intended, genetic mother must legally adopt her own baby. In other states, motherhood is determined by genetics. In yet a third group of states, maternity is determined by contract. Would-be parents in the United States, therefore, must navigate a complex legal journey, while simultaneously making their way through a multifaceted emotional and medical maze.

Surrogacy arrangements, while a seemingly modern approach to bringing a baby into the world, are not exactly a new development. The Old Testament references Hagar, maid to Sarah, bearing a child for Sarah and Abraham when Sarah was unable to do so. A couple of hundred years later, in Babylonian times, King Hammurabi promulgated the Hammurabi Code of Laws, setting out the rules of the day. Among them: "A childless wife might give her husband a maid (who was no wife) to bear him children, who were reckoned hers."[1] A fairly clear endorsement of traditional surrogacy. The development of IVF enabled the evolution of the relatively less complicated gestational surrogacy, in which the surrogate mother, or host, is not related to the baby she is carrying for the intended parents. Since its first successful, healthy birth in 1985, gestational surrogacy has become the norm for women experiencing infertility or repeat miscarriage, eliminating the need for a traditional surrogate to give up her own biological child.[2]

Although surrogacy has been practiced for millennia, the complicated moral and ethical issues involved in surrogacy arrangements—particularly commercial surrogacy in which the "consumers" are often well-off intended parents and the surrogates typically far less affluent—seem to have paralyzed American lawmakers, who, by and large, have left the issue untouched. Does it make sense, for example, that one can buy eggs or sperm on the Internet in the same states where gestational surrogacy is prohibited?

In contrast, in most developed countries, surrogacy is regulated by national governments, with legislation ranging from outright bans to clear requirements.[3] In the United Kingdom, Ireland, Denmark, and Belgium, for example, surrogacy is permitted but commercial (paid) surrogacy is not; in Israel, while restricted to those who meet certain criteria (i.e., heterosexual couples only, the intended parents and surrogate must practice the same religion, the surrogate must be single, the semen must be that of the husband and not a donor), gestational surrogacy is funded in totality by the state, and the birth mother does not have any legal status with respect to the baby. France, Germany, Italy, Spain, and Portugal, among others, forbid all forms of surrogacy. It is essential for a third-party parent-to-be to get fully educated on the legal ramifications of undergoing a treatment in a particular jurisdiction.

In the United States, the laws vary wildly by state, and not always along the lines you might expect. California, Arkansas, Illinois, and Tennessee are among the best jurisdictions for gestational surrogacy, while New York, Arizona, Nebraska, Michigan, Louisiana, and Washington, DC, are among the worst. In Michigan, for instance, individuals who enter into surrogacy contracts can be fined up to $50,000 and imprisoned for up to five years; Washington, DC, similarly, imposes fines of up to $10,000, a prison sentence of up to one year, or both.[4] New

York forbids paid gestational surrogacy, although New York State senator Brad Hoylman, father of a child born through a surrogate, is cosponsor of a bill called the Child-Parent Security Act, a proposed law that would overturn the current law and make compensated surrogacy legal in New York State.[5] Neighboring New Jersey permits it (although the courts will not necessarily enforce surrogacy contracts). So, naturally, there is a burgeoning business of would-be parents being treated at clinics in New York crossing the Hudson on the day of embryo transfer (particularly if the surrogate does not live in New Jersey), as we did in our failed attempt with Brenda, or traveling to nearby Connecticut or Pennsylvania, where they pay yet another clinic to transfer their embryos into a surrogate.

More confusing still, most states have no clear laws on the books. In Alaska, Colorado, Connecticut, Georgia, Hawaii, and nearly two dozen other states, in the absence of explicit laws, courts are often favorable to intended parents, although there is no guarantee—a large risk to take with respect to custody of your child. Legal expert Melissa Brisman believes it is in the best interests of all involved for states to enact clear laws specifying that intended parents are legally responsible for the children that they create. Responding to the fact that most people are worried about what happens if a surrogate wants to keep a baby, Brisman points out the flip side of that coin. "What if the baby is born with a defect, and the intended parents decide they don't want to take responsibility? You have the surrogate, who gave this wonderful gift, and now she's stuck with parental rights and responsibilities."[6] Sean Tipton, chief advocacy, policy, and development officer of the American Society for Reproductive Medicine (ASRM), does not disagree, claiming that fertility specialists would welcome thoughtful attempts to clarify parentage laws, "making it clear what parental rights and obligations are, and how to obtain or relinquish them."[7]

Despite the challenges, increasing numbers of hopeful parents are turning to surrogacy to build their families. And while not every surrogate birth goes as smoothly as Alexandra's—reflective to some extent of the fact that not all births go as well, and not all hospitals as indulgent— virtually everyone with whom I spoke who became a parent via surrogacy had an extremely positive, albeit sometimes stressful, surrogate experience.

When Robert and Jeffrey, a same-sex couple who are both medical professionals in DC, decided to have a baby with a surrogate and egg donor, they desired professional guidance and support, and went straight to an established agency. In choosing their surrogate, they were concerned primarily with health and a good fit for their family rather than proximity. They didn't mind that she lived in Ohio and they would not see her regularly, although they did travel to be with her for all the milestones. Their surrogate pregnancies went extremely smoothly, and they felt tremendous joy and gratitude at the birth of their daughter, and later twin boys, born of the same surrogate, who remains a special family friend.

Paula, to the contrary, wanted a surrogate nearby, close enough to be able to participate in the appointments. Convinced after her fifth miscarriage and further diagnoses that she could not carry a child, Paula, like me, was determined to find her own surrogate. When her first two choices didn't work out for various reasons, she eventually turned to an agency in her hometown and happily found a surrogate not too far away. Their proximity proved fortuitous, as Paula and Derrick were awakened one night at 3:00 a.m. and rushed to the hospital upon learning that their surrogate, Amy, was in labor at only twenty-six weeks and four days. In addition to their overwhelming fear for the health of their twin babies, who were each born weighing less than two pounds and were immediately rushed into incubators, they worried about Amy and the impact on her husband and her son, struggling with the guilt of knowing that Amy had put her health and her family at risk for them. Paula and Derrick felt tremendous relief when they learned that Amy was OK—though the guilt persisted. Paula felt that she should have been experiencing the difficulty and pain instead of their surrogate.

Similarly, Pietro and Peter, professional dancers living in Houston, experienced the full gamut of emotions. From gratitude and wonder to disappointment, guilt, and helplessness. From the outset, they felt strongly about working with an agency and surrogate who were local so they could participate in every aspect of the pregnancy. Their relationship with their first surrogate fell apart because she decided she no longer felt comfortable working with a gay couple. Her withdrawal left Pietro and Peter so shattered that it made them take a step back and reconsider the whole process. "We weren't feeling as confident," Pietro, who is from Italy, explained. They felt let down by both the surrogate and the agency, who had assured them that she was happy to work with them.

Longing for a child, they eventually found the strength to try again. Working with a different, more experienced agency, they quickly narrowed their search to two potential surrogates. After meeting the surrogates in person, they felt a good connection with one: twenty-one years old and with one daughter, she was inspired by seeing two of her good friends serve as surrogates for others, and quickly agreed to work with them. Although she didn't struggle at all emotionally, as is often a concern for intended parents, she had a very hard time physically. She didn't feel well from the time she started the hormone shots and continued to feel poorly throughout the pregnancy. She started spotting at fifteen weeks, and after a very stressful few weeks, sadly lost the baby in the eighteenth week. She eventually had a D&C, and Peter and Pietro learned, to their great surprise, that the fetus was fine, with the normal complement of chromosomes.

Devastated by the loss, they didn't discuss it for a year, until a call from the embryo bank regarding its storage fee reopened the conversation. Soon after, their agency found a new surrogate for them—an American woman married to an Italian with whom she shared two daughters. From the moment they met Cindy, they knew they had found the all-important perfect fit. The IVF went smoothly, and Cindy became pregnant with twins. At fifteen weeks, the heartbeat of one stopped, causing them to relive the trauma of their first loss. Pietro had upsetting dreams in which he saw his dead baby lying next to his live baby. As they mourned, Cindy, still pregnant with the other twin, was a great source of optimism and stability. Later in the pregnancy, the baby's placenta stuck to Cindy's uterine wall, causing bleeding and putting her health at risk. Cindy went in for a necessary C-section six weeks early and gave birth to a beautiful baby girl, but the placenta had burrowed too far into her uterus, causing her to have an unplanned hysterectomy (thankfully covered by insurance they had purchased), which Pietro regrets to this day.

Naturally, sometimes, as with all pregnancies, surrogates miscarry, which is crushing for all involved. After seven miscarriages, Jessica and Ethan had turned to surrogacy as their last hope. Jessica found her own surrogate, who had successfully given birth to three babies, and they began the process at the clinic she had grown to hate; she was willing to try just about anything to have the baby they longed for. Emma, their surrogate, conceived on the first try, and both the pregnancy and their relationship progressed beautifully. In her second trimester, Emma miscarried. Their "sure thing" had failed them. Jessica's words at the time so eloquently convey the depth of her devastation: "I hurt. Not in a scary way, not in a can't-get-out-of-bed way. But in a can't-stop-crying way. I imagine my heart dripping down into my stomach and slipping out of my body in a sea of tears. If my heart melted away, maybe I would hurt less. I have come to love and hate hope. I want to disown hope, that horrible tease of an emotion, so I can just be peacefully numb for a bit. A welcome reprieve."

When it works, surrogacy can be a win-win for all, not only enabling the birth of a much-desired child, but often, in the process, creating unexpected, sometimes lifelong bonds. Sitting in Robert and Jeffrey's kitchen on a rainy Sunday morning in DC, drinking coffee with their surrogate, Jo, and her friend, who were visiting from Ohio, I was struck by both the beauty and the normalcy of the scene. Three happy, giggling children playing in the background, while their two dads and surrogate who carried them chatted with me about their unconventional family. Jo was so moved by the experience, she switched careers and began working for the surrogate agency that had connected them. While accustomed to hearing parents rave about the surrogates who carried their children, it was Jo's response about their surrogacy journey that stayed with me verbatim: "It was a privilege and a joy."

Alone we can do so little; together we can do so much.

Helen Keller

When It Takes a Village

Surrogacy and Egg Donation

Twenty months on, Alexandra's birth still seemed like a miracle. She was walking (sort of) and talking (often in words only I could understand). Yet it was harder to give up on trying for Number Two than I expected. We had been trying to have a baby for more than six years, and it had become part of my daily life. After the failure of the agreed-upon "last IVF cycle ever," my acquiescence to finally getting off the IVF treadmill was helped along by our big international move. Richard had accepted a job in Dubai and had been commuting there from London for six months, partly because I insisted he make sure that he liked it before we uprooted our small family and left a city we loved, but also so that I could continue my fertility treatments. With the latter constraint now sadly out of the picture, and Richard enjoying his job and Dubai, I arranged—not without difficulty and drama, of course—to transfer to my law firm's new Abu Dhabi office. It sounded logistically easy to me at the time, as Abu Dhabi, the capital of the United Arab Emirates, was just sixty-odd miles away from Dubai. Maps don't let you know that the route between the two cities is a death-defying road across a desert, where car pileups reach into double and triple digits.

Richard and I set off for the Emirates with Alexandra; our cat, Sesame; and, for the first time in years, no goal of family expansion. We would enjoy our daughter and our time in the sun, taking some time to process what we had been through. Maybe we would adopt in the future. Maybe we would be "one and done."

It didn't take very long to adjust to life in what felt like an episode of *The Jetsons*. We met new friends from all over the world and experienced the incredible buzz that was Dubai before the financial crash. It was far enough removed from our everyday lives that shots and IVF and PGS receded quickly into the past—until my phone started to ring. My friend Andrea had a friend Alice, in London, who had cancer and needed some advice on egg and embryo freezing and surrogacy, and my friend Olga had a friend Michelle, from New Zealand, who lived in Moscow and was desperate to talk to me about IVF protocols. Sarah, a college friend now living in New York, had a friend who needed advice as well. Friends and acquaintances of my mother began to call, all desperate to help their fertility-challenged daughters or daughters-in-law.

I spoke to Michelle, the New Zealander in Moscow, at length about IVF and miscarriage. She asked me why I hadn't considered treatment in Russia or Ukraine, particularly since I had worked and lived in Moscow on and off while trying to conceive. Russia or Ukraine? They were not on my radar screen. But Michelle told me that Russia and Ukraine, along with Israel, had among the highest success rates in the world. She gave me the names of the clinics she was considering and sent me all the information she had assembled. The numbers were unbelievable— I mean really unbelievable. It couldn't be true. Nearly a 70 percent live birth rate at her top two choices—in contrast with an average of approximately 30 percent in the United States and 25 percent in the

United Kingdom across all age groups in 2011. She went for an appointment at the AltraVita clinic in Moscow and was impressed. Then forty-three years old, Michelle had somehow endured thirteen miscarriages and was focusing on adoption. Yet after her visit to the clinic, she decided to try IVF one more time. Her protocol was totally different from those I had seen before—partly because many of the hormones had different brand names, but also because the dosages and duration were shorter, and there were a number of items on the list that I had never heard of. She became pregnant with twins. Everyone she met going through the cycle at that clinic also became pregnant. She urged me to go see her doctor.

I was torn. We had a wonderful daughter and had put much of our pain and anguish behind us. We had had our hopes raised and crushed so many times. I didn't want to put either of us through that emotional turmoil again. But I also kept thinking about a conversation with my cousin Caryn at our farewell gathering in New York as we were embarking on our move to Dubai. A sister and a mother of three, she had taken me aside and urged me not to give up on trying to get a sibling for Alexandra. And I couldn't imagine my own life without my brother.

Fortuitously, a business trip to Moscow came up. I convinced myself it was fate. I called the Moscow clinic and begged for an appointment during my two-day visit. After several back-and-forths, the English speaker at the other end of the phone finally scheduled a consultation for me during one of the doctor's lunch breaks. Richard agreed to the consultation, but he was not willing to commit to anything else. Although we had quietly, and somewhat uneasily, discussed the option of IVF with an egg donor, for the most part it had remained on the back burner as Richard had simply had enough of the fertility drama.

Other than our good friends Jeff and Olga, who kindly put us up during our treatment visits, we didn't tell anyone—including my mother—about that first trip. Or any of the trips that followed. Having now turned forty, even I knew that it looked like I had finally lost my marbles.

I went straight to the clinic from the airport, with my carry-on bag and a healthy dose of skepticism measured by a touch of new hope. Dr. Oxana sat in front of me with my file on her desk, her inscrutable face skimming her Russian notes for what seemed like a very long time. She finally spoke, through the translator. "OK, first you do tests, next we decide how we proceed."

I turned to look at the translator. "But I have a number of questions before I decide if I even want to proceed."

"What questions?"

"Does the doctor really think it makes sense," I asked, "for me to try again? Would I need an egg donor? I don't seem to have any good eggs."

The translator spoke, and the doctor smiled as she replied, her warm brown eyes softening. "You wouldn't know if you had any good eggs. The high level of drugs would have ruined them. You may have several."

Dr. Oxana explained her plan. First, I would follow a homeopathic detox regime to help rid my body of the hormones I had pumped into myself during my multiple IVF treatments in New York and London; she insisted that the damaging levels of hormones in my body were compromising my egg quality. Then, once I was detoxed, I would begin IVF, on a short protocol, at a very low level of drugs. When I started to express my concern that there wouldn't be any eggs to retrieve at those dosages, she became frustrated. Either I accepted the clinic's philosophy or I didn't, she explained. It was very simple.

Accept her *philosophy*? Whoever heard of an IVF philosophy? Dr. Oxana told me with little fanfare (through her translator) that the doctors in Russia had a different philosophy from those in the United States. In the West, she explained, most doctors believe that the chromosomal health of a woman's eggs is essentially determined at birth and degrades with age, and that it is the job of the fertility specialist to coax out the highest number of eggs to find the "healthy" ones, i.e., the proverbial needle-in-the-haystack approach. In contrast, in Russia (and Ukraine and certain clinics in Israel, Japan, and Western Europe, among others), she explained, many fertility specialists believe that the environment in the body, and in the outside world, greatly affects the health of the eggs and thus the embryos produced; that diet, toxins, chemicals, hormones—especially of high dosage as in the very IVF protocols I had been following—potentially *harmed* the eggs I was so desperately trying to harvest. Rather than stimulating the production of as many eggs as possible in an assumption that it would increase the chances of finding at least one good one, Dr. Oxana was seeking to gently stimulate the production of only a handful of eggs, hoping to find one or two good ones.

She and her colleagues also believe, radically, that egg quality can be improved. Not only is egg quality not static, it can go up as well as down. "At six hundred units of Puregon [the amount taken during my last cycle in New York], all your eggs would be damaged," Dr. Oxana said. "I will use one hundred and fifty to two hundred and fifty units. We will probably have only four eggs, but half should be normal. That is all you need."

All your eggs would be damaged. Could this be true? That's all I could hear. After all I had been through, how could I not know this? Could the basic premise of five torturous, expensive, and sad years' worth of IVF— the very cornerstone of Western medical reproductive orthodoxy—be wrong? I could still have good eggs? Or I could get them again?

If it were true, in addition to increasing the chance of conception, her approach would also potentially increase the odds of keeping the pregnancy. Given that chromosomal abnormalities, which cause more miscarriages than all other known causes of miscarriage combined, most often result from an abnormal egg, could we have been doing something more effective all along not only to conceive but also to help prevent the miscarriages? These are the questions that would haunt me, and drive me, from that moment on.

Dr. Oxana explained that her detox plan—comprising a number of homeopathic remedies from a German company named Heel, together with the necessary daily multivitamins and the elimination of all plastics (bottles, containers, Tupperware) from my life—was designed to rid my body of its high level of toxins, creating a healthy environment for the growth of my eggs. The low dose hormone protocol was intended to minimize any damage from the current IVF cycle. Her goal: to stimulate healthy eggs using the least invasive means possible.

We began a complex negotiation, the Russian doctor and the American lawyer.

"Your eggs, use surrogate."

"Donor eggs, carry myself."

A standoff.

Dr. Oxana was absolutely insistent that my own eggs would work with her regime. But I was skeptical of her plan—doctors I had trusted believed I had *no good eggs left,* and I had certainly never heard of improving egg quality—so I pushed to use donor eggs, despite my continued unease, as backup.

As for my carrying the baby, however, Dr. Oxana had concerns. She was very worried about possible immunological and anatomical challenges to my carrying to term. She felt that my antiphospholipid syndrome and elevated natural killer cells posed significant risks, and she also worried about the unusual shape of my uterus. She explained that embryos would prefer to implant in a nicely shaped uterus with a smooth surface, and my arcuate or septate (irregularly shaped, almost bifurcated) uterus did not present the most welcoming environment. She seemed somewhat irritated that my file contained virtually no information on the shape of my uterus, the sole letter regarding my HSG test the only evidence they had ever looked at it. She said my uterus "did not make her feel good" about my prospects for implantation, and urged me to use a surrogate to protect against miscarriage.

She admittedly had good points, especially with regard to my carrying. Yet she couldn't sway me. Intoxicated with the idea that all my miscarriages may have been due to poor egg and therefore poor embryo quality, I felt there was no reason I shouldn't be able to carry myself with good eggs—someone else's good eggs, that is. And as much as I wanted to believe her and felt tantalized by the prospect of my own bio-logical child, I just couldn't get my head around the idea that she could find good eggs in me, at age forty, when every doctor, embryologist, nurse, ob-gyn, and article I had ever read assured me that my aging eggs were no longer viable.

We compromised, agreeing to proceed, unusually, with a dual cycle: a donor and I would both go through the egg stimulation proto-col at the same time, and we would select the best quality embryos to transfer to me to carry.

Managing the cycle was, admittedly, a little more complex than the others, and believe me, I was used to complexity. Dr. Oxana was in Moscow, I lived in Dubai, and I had to obtain specialized products from Germany. She started out by requiring me to follow her detox plan for forty days, and we made an appointment for my return visit for blood tests. Fortunately, the flight from Dubai to Moscow was only three hours, and I could do it as an overnight trip, but it was a heck of a long way to go for a blood test. Seven weeks later, I was back in her office. The nurse drew my blood. I waited. I saw Dr. Oxana for about three minutes. She told me I wasn't ready. Forty more days. I flew back home. Repeat.

While on Dr. Oxana's homeopathic detox protocol, I studied lists of potential egg donors: height, weight, hair color, eye color, face shape, blood type. Per Russian law, no photos were allowed. I pre-sented the contenders to Richard. The trick was to try to imagine a girl in Russia who looked like me, which actually wasn't too hard, since I am largely of Russian Jewish descent. The woman who man-aged the list at the clinic was outspoken and opinionated, but also helpful. I e-mailed Katya, the translator, to enquire about a few candi-date numbers (the women were nameless, of course) and her answers never failed to crack a smile. "She is a fine donor, but looks nothing like you." "She is a nice girl, but I am not sure if you would be happy." That one intrigued me. She told me later that she wasn't very bright, "certainly not suitable for a lawyer."

Selecting an egg donor is like holding a mirror up to yourself and wondering what you might choose to see if you had the power to change things. Did I want an egg donor who was taller? Or exactly my height? With my color eyes, or perhaps bright blue? Blond or brunette? Someone athletic? Well educated? Had a career? The choices never stop. The process forced me, somewhat uncomfortably, to confront what mattered to me in choosing the genetic material for my child. And then, it overwhelmed me. Uncomfortable with the role of creator, I simply deferred to my clinic, as Dr. Oxana had originally suggested we do. Katya e-mailed to tell me that a donor had come in who looked remarkably like me, and the coordinator thought she was a perfect fit. Done. Uncomfortable choices avoided.

As luck would have it, by the time I was ready to begin the IVF cycle, I had found the perfect doctor in Dubai who was willing to work directly with Dr. Oxana. Dr. Nataliya, a Bulgarian ob-gyn who had recently moved to Dubai, came highly recommended from friends, and it was an unexpected blessing that she spoke Russian and was somewhat familiar with treatment there. We worked out an effective, albeit time-consuming, system. I went to the Cooper Health Clinic every other day, where I had acupuncture treatments from her Australian colleague Martine, and saw Dr. Nataliya for blood tests and ultrasound scans. She would then e-mail the results to Moscow, and I would go down to the sun-filled waiting room, get a cup of green tea, and happily begin my perusal of fashion and gossip magazines. At some point within the next hour or two, she would receive a return e-mail from AltraVita with our daily instructions, which she would relay to me in English.

One sunny afternoon, much like all the others, Dr. Nataliya announced that there was good news. I was to go to Moscow the next day for egg retrieval. It happened to be my birthday, and so, rather than celebrating by going to the Coldplay concert in Dubai as originally planned, Richard and I gave the much coveted tickets to some delighted friends and flew to Moscow to see if Dr. Oxana's theory about egg rejuvenation would bear fruit.

As it turned out, Dr. Oxana was right about everything. After nearly three months of following her every instruction, she retrieved eight eggs (which she thought was too many, although I was thrilled), which in turn produced four embryos, two of which were normal (as revealed by preimplantation genetic testing). After several rounds of precisely zero normal embryos, and our earlier results of only one out of eight and three out of thirteen normals, I was both shocked and thrilled to have *50 percent* of my embryos turn out to be chromosomally normal. Although she advised me that one of the two did not look good, I desperately wanted to use my own embryos, rather than those of the twenty-one-year-old donor I had been reluctantly relying on. With dwindling minutes for debate, the doctor pushed me into transferring one of each. An experienced hand at egg donation, she was sure I would get pregnant, and was also sure it wouldn't matter to me at all in the end whose egg it was once I had a healthy baby in my arms. Filled with anxiety, I acquiesced. Or rather, I didn't object as they swiftly rolled me away and she firmly instructed the team in Russian. In reality, it happened so quickly, I didn't have much say in the matter.

When I first found out I was pregnant, after transferring one of my own embryos and one of my donor's, my initial reaction was shock. I was happy, of course, that we had two good embryos to transfer (both male, they revealed after the fact), and, unlike with my last several pregnancies, hopeful that I would finally keep one. At the same time, much to my surprise, I began to dwell on the fact that I had one of each inside me, and wondered if it was a mistake not to have transferred two of my own embryos. I realized only then that I hadn't thought through the donor question as thoroughly as I should have, and hadn't truly made my peace with using someone else's egg. I found it ironic that the ethics committee at the Lister Fertility Clinic, which forbade surrogacy, a temporary relationship, had no problem whatsoever allowing for and facilitating egg donation, a very permanent one. It just seemed backward to me. As opposed to serving as a lovely, living breathing "oven," this generous, anonymous woman would potentially provide the genetic basis of our child.

In my panic, I tried to figure out how I got here. We had previously ruled out egg donation when we thought we needed a surrogate. Unlike the thousands of people who turn to egg donation each year in hopes of having a healthy child, for me, the idea of needing both an egg donor and a surrogate felt a step too far. If I couldn't carry the baby, and the baby would not contain my genetic material, then I couldn't see why we should go to all this trouble to create a baby when there were real, live babies who needed homes. But everything changed so swiftly when, at the ripe old age of forty, Dr. Oxana told me that she suspected I had good eggs. Excited about the chance of trying again to have my own child, and perhaps even carry the pregnancy this time, I had argued for the donor backup plan because I simply couldn't face going through yet another IVF cycle only to come up empty-handed. But it was really just that: a plan I was trying to make as airtight as possible. My thought process went no further than the mechanics of ensuring that we had some good eggs to transfer. I certainly hadn't contemplated the possibility of transferring a mixed batch.

Despite our lack of a common language, Dr. Oxana always read my face.

"Relax," she reprimanded me, "it doesn't matter."

"But I won't know if the baby is genetically mine, or the donor's."

"And it doesn't matter. When you hold the baby in your arms, you will understand that it doesn't matter." I wanted to believe her, but I worried. Should we genetically test the baby and find out? Would it be strange if my daughter was genetically mine and my son was not? Would he be jealous? Closer to his father? What if, against the odds, both had implanted and we were having half-blood twins? Did it matter? Richard did not seem to think it mattered. Nor, clearly, did Dr. Oxana or Katya, the only other people who knew our unique situation.

A few weeks later, when I lost our (one) baby, I was too sad for tears. My seventh miscarriage was no less devastating than the six that had been definitively "mine."

Life continued on in Dubai, but I couldn't stop thinking about our experience at AltraVita. Dr. Oxana had been right about the eggs. Why had I been so stubborn about carrying myself? If I hadn't, we might be expecting another child now. I thought I had made my peace with having no more biological children, believing it was a closed door, but Dr. Oxana had cracked the door open and a sliver of light now shone in. I had produced two normal, healthy embryos. Surely she could get more? I knew I had to try. Dr. Oxana remained optimistic but insisted that we use a surrogate if we were to try again with her. This time, I didn't argue.

With Catherine, our "practically perfect" surrogate, as we had fondly come to call her, sadly out of the picture, I was back to square one. I met with a Russian law firm and surrogacy agency. I looked online again at the various surrogacy sites. I studied India and Ukraine as options, contacting clinics there and poring over their databases. I corresponded with several women. And then one evening, in Dubai, my phone rang. Catherine had news. She had broken up with Paul, her fiancé. She offered to try one last time for us. Our fairy godmother.

The protocol remained much the same. In fact, even lower dose, as Dr. Oxana reduced the Gonal-f from 250 IU per day as used in the first cycle to 150 IU the second time because, ironically, she thought I had produced too many eggs. I was back to Dr. Nataliya and Martine for monitoring and acupuncture. I brushed up on my celebrity gossip in the lobby while awaiting my daily call.

Richard and I went to Russia in July 2009. I took several days off work, promising to be available by phone, and we left Alexandra in Dubai in the care of dear friends. It was a frantically rushed trip. Despite my careful planning, I had failed to digest the key fact that it was illegal in Russia for a surrogate to be thirty-five or older, and Catherine's thirty-fifth birthday was on July 11. If our embryos were not transferred to her by July 10, it was over. My eggs, thankfully, were retrieved on the Fourth of July. The procedure was smooth, and Dr. Oxana retrieved seven eggs, which were promptly fertilized and resulted in four embryos. His part done, Richard returned to Dubai, where work and Alexandra awaited.

Catherine arrived a couple of days later, just as the embryologist was doing the embryo biopsy for PGS. I suppressed my anxiety about having good embryos to transfer, somewhat fearful that Catherine would be annoyed, at best, that we had dragged her to Moscow when we were uncertain of even having our own embryos to transfer; on top of that, I hadn't dared broach the idea of her carrying a donor's embryo. I think I had been hoping for the best and ignoring the worst. But now I was pacing around my hotel room wondering how I had let Dr. Oxana talk me into such a low dosage. I had never had so few eggs to start with. I convinced myself there would be nothing left.

Finally, Katya, the translator, called. All four embryos were chromosomally normal. *One hundred percent*. I was speechless. Three boys and a girl. What a contrast to my last two attempts with the traditional protocol, which had yielded the devastating result of nice-looking embryos, all of which were chromosomally abnormal, many rife with complex abnormalities. Now, having crossed the dreaded forty-year-old milestone, I had virtually the same result as my fertile young donor!

Remarkably, the sun shone down on us as we toured around Moscow, Red Square, the Kremlin, GUM. We dined at the elegant Café Pushkin, where I was allowed my first drink as Catherine had her last. I barely slept that night, tossing, turning, and praying my embryos would not arrest overnight.

Catherine and I awoke on July 9, two days before her thirty-fifth birthday, and promptly got into a taxi to take us from the Golden Apple Boutique Hotel off Tverskaya in central Moscow out to the AltraVita clinic. The taxi picked up speed after we left the halting bustle of the city, and as we glided along the highway I turned to smile at Catherine.

Despite having done this before, we were both nervous, but my excitement was mounting too. This might well be the time that we got it right. There was no reason to think otherwise. Suddenly, unbelievably, our taxi rammed into the truck ahead of us and jolted to a halt. I started speaking to the driver in panicked, halting Russian, which he could not understand. Despite our lack of communication, one thing was clear: his car was not going to AltraVita that morning. Standing in the tiny shoulder of the highway with tears in my eyes, I felt a crazy panic threatening to take over. The embryologist would be preparing the embryos now, and I needed to get to that clinic. I called my friend Olga, and in a mad jumble of words somehow managed to convey that I needed her to talk to the driver and ask him how we could get to the clinic. He told her there was no way, but he did manage to describe where we were. Olga agreed that she would send a car, but with Moscow traffic, it could take an hour for the car to get to us, let alone get to the clinic. Just as my heart was starting to slow down enough for me to realize that it had been racing, a taxi passed by and the driver shouted at me in Russian. I held out the cell phone and he hit the brakes. Olga must have explained where we needed to go, because next thing I knew, we were in the back of a filthy black tinted Lada. But it moved, and I was grateful. We arrived, frazzled, an hour late to the clinic.

Rushing to get Catherine ready for the transfer, the Russian nurse whisked her away before I could speak to anyone. Dr. Oxana emerged eventually and spoke to me in English. "Congratulations," she said. She had transferred the best-looking embryos, which happened to be two boys, to Catherine, and sent our healthy girl (the third boy didn't make it), along with our donor embryos, to the freezer (where they remain to this day).

"Good luck with the pregnancy," she said with a smile.

Katya then led me upstairs into a room where a cameraman and reporter awaited me. I was totally confused.

"I thought they asked your permission," Katya murmured, surprised by my reaction.

"They did," I replied. "In theory. I thought they might call me some-day to be interviewed in a TV studio, with hair and makeup and lighting."

She laughed, but I wasn't joking.

"I am not only a mess, I am not prepared," I protested, as a lawyer used to preparing for every meeting.

"Not prepared?" Katya laughed. "You have been preparing for nine years."

Unkempt, exhausted, and nervous, I spoke to the CNN International crew. They had interviewed patients from all over the world who had come to Russia, virtually all of whom had had success, some after as many as a dozen miscarriages, but I was the first American they had an opportunity to meet. The show would air on CNN International, they informed me, on *Connect the World* with Becky Anderson, but they weren't sure if they could get it onto CNN in America. In any event, they wanted others to hear the perspective of an American who sought treatment in Russia. It was a fraught, yet important ending to a fraught, yet important day.

Unfortunately for Catherine, her second surrogate pregnancy was tougher than the first. She had morning sickness for much of the pregnancy, and was just miserable. I felt terrible every time I spoke with her on the phone. The guilt was overwhelming. She was suffering so much to give us a baby, and there was not a darn thing we could do to make her feel better. The distance was tougher on all of us too. Living in Dubai, with Catherine in England, we couldn't participate the way we had with Alexandra and couldn't support her as much as we would have liked. Thankfully, she had her wonderful family to help out, accompanying her to appointments with the doctor and staying with her when she was ill. We spoke and e-mailed frequently, of course, and I flew to England to accompany her to all the big milestone examinations, but we missed out on the others. I was incredibly grateful we had established such a strong relationship during her first surrogate pregnancy. It would have been all the more difficult if this were the first.

On the evening of March 9, 2010, about three weeks before our due date, I was in my bedroom in Dubai, having just put Alexandra to bed, when my phone rang. Catherine had preeclampsia and her blood pressure had gotten dangerously high. They were planning to induce labor. How soon could we get there? Within two hours, Richard and I were at the airport with a very heavy-eyed Alexandra and haphazardly packed bags. We took a red-eye to London, rented a car, and started driving to the hospital. When I turned my phone back on after the flight, my voice-mail box was full. Catherine gave birth to a very squishy, yellow, sleepy baby just as our wheels hit the ground at Heathrow. He was induced so strongly he literally shot through the birth canal. We raced to the hospital. Drowsy and confused, Alexandra asked where we were as we walked through the doors of the maternity ward.

"Darling," I answered, "meet your baby brother, William."

"And please give a hug to favorite Auntie Catherine," Catherine chimed in from her bed.

"Yes, Alexandra. Say hello to favorite Auntie Catherine." I smiled. That's Alexandra's nickname for Catherine. I call her Catherine the Great.

Egg and Sperm Donation

As with surrogacy, many aspects of egg, sperm, and embryo donation are legal and policy minefields. While certain medical aspects of donation are regulated nationally by the US Food and Drug Administration (FDA), complex issues such as donor compensation, anonymity, and the right of children to seek out the identity of their biological parent after they are eighteen remain outside the sphere of regulation, varying from state to state and clinic to clinic. Intended parents using donor sperm or egg, unlike those working with surrogates, fortunately do not have to face the terrifying question of whether their baby will be legally recognized as their own. But they face other obstacles, as regulations surrounding donation have simply not caught up with the scientific advances or the ethical questions. Neither the federal nor state governments, for example, regulate how many children may be conceived from one sperm donor; although the American Society for Reproductive Medicine suggests a limit of twenty-five births per population area of eight hundred thousand, there are reported cases of donors fathering sixty, seventy, one hundred, and even one hundred and fifty offspring.[1] Nor do they regulate the age range in which an egg or sperm donor must fall; the type of medical information donors must provide, apart from an FDA requirement to test for infectious diseases, such as HIV; or whether the children conceived as a result of donation have any right to know of their origins. In contrast with the United Kingdom, in which the Human Fertilisation and Embryology Authority tracks all donor births, and many other developed countries that have followed the British regulatory model, in the United States, there is no central registry for donor-conceived children.[2]

These are thorny questions with real-life implications. If a man in a small town donates sperm regularly, what is to stop two children from unknowingly falling in love and committing "accidental incest"—a genuine concern when donors can father upward of one hundred half siblings? If he has a genetic disorder, such as sickle cell anemia or cystic fibrosis, or a predisposition to heart defects or schizophrenia, to how many children will the disorder unknowingly be passed on? There are hundreds of known cases of genetic defects being passed from donor to child, and experts believe there could be thousands. In one sibling group from the same donor, there are at least eight children with a deadly heart defect, and as many as three dozen born of a donor with mental illness.[3] Is it fair that children conceived of donor eggs or sperm may have no knowledge of their own medical histories if their parents choose not to tell them how they were conceived?

To date, such questions are addressed on an ad hoc basis by local laws and courts, as is the controversy regarding donor compensation, particularly with respect to egg donation, which is significantly more intrusive and complicated than sperm donation. How much is enough for a woman willing to undergo weeks of hormone injections, blood tests, invasive ultrasound examinations, and egg retrieval, as well as expose herself to potential health risks, in order to help someone else have a baby? How much is too much, creating the feeling (or possibility) that a woman is selling her eggs like a commodity? Are advertisements in newspapers and on subways, college campuses, and Facebook offering compensation for giving the "gift of life" coercive, or troubling in light of the possibility that high levels of hormones taken in a typical conventional IVF cycle may have negative consequences for repeat donors, a topic that requires far more research?

In the United States, the pricing of eggs and sperm, like other issues surrounding fertility, is largely driven by the marketplace. Most states have yet to delve into these issues, and to the extent that states have enacted regulations, such as with surrogacy, they often conflict with one another.

In contrast, a number of developed countries, including much of Western Europe, Canada, and Australia, have confronted these issues head-on. Italy and Switzerland, for example, prohibit egg and sperm donation as well as surrogacy. Australia, Belgium, Canada, the Netherlands, and the United Kingdom permit these practices but prohibit the commercial purchase of donor eggs and sperm. Spain and the United Kingdom have limited the number of children that can be born from a single sperm donor to six and ten, respectively. Japan's laws puzzlingly conflict with themselves: a donor of eggs or sperm has a right to anonymity, while a child born of a donated egg, upon reaching the age of fifteen, has a right to know his or her origins.[4] The United Kingdom, Austria, Finland, Germany, the Netherlands, New Zealand, Norway, Sweden, Switzerland, and certain parts of Australia allow donation but prohibit donor anonymity, in the belief that children have a right to know their genetic heritage.[5]

These are choppy waters to navigate. In the United States, where there is no requirement to tell children of their origins, views among parents, practitioners, and family therapists vary widely. Parents in heterosexual couples face the threshold question of whether to tell their children of the existence of a donor. Advocates of the "tell" side rely on the most obvious of arguments: truth, maintaining that not only do the children of donors have a right to know the truth, but also, pragmatically, that truth will in all likelihood come out in the end, especially with the increasing availability of DNA testing. Most family therapists support openness and honesty within the family, as does, officially, the American Society for Reproductive Medicine, although the ASRM, like many doctors, does not aggressively push that position. Perhaps recognizing the reality that more than half of potential patients are leaning toward nondisclosure,[6] these clinicians may have a fear of alienating clients.

The reasons parents, especially women, offer for not telling their children cover a broader spectrum, although the response I most often received to the question was along the lines of "I'm not sure why exactly . . . I'm just not comfortable with it." According to Joan Manheimer, a clinical psychologist at the University of Colorado Advanced Reproductive Medicine specializing in fertility, moving on to egg donation is often, for women who have failed to give birth, the most difficult aspect of negotiating the rocky infertility road. Discussing the emotional trauma some women with infertility experience, Dr. Manheimer explained that many women are initially "shocked to find out that they have a problem because it doesn't fit with how they feel." They often then experience what she calls an "undefined loss."[7] There is no physical loss to grieve; rather they grieve the loss of having the genetic baby they had always assumed they would have.

Some women process that loss and are ready to move on in the open. Others are perhaps ashamed of being infertile, a condition that they fear may be stigmatized in our society. One woman, who did not want to be quoted, said she feared her parents would not accept the baby as their own grandchild; another said she thought that telling "wasn't important" and would only make her child feel different or hurt. Patricia Mendell, a therapist who specializes in reproductive issues, finds that one of the most poignant reasons women or couples find it hard to come clean is that they get caught up in the fairy-tale version of the "perfect" baby in a "normal" family, convincing themselves that "it's better for the child not to know the truth."[8] Barry Stevens, maker of the documentary *Offspring* about his search for his biological father, begs to differ: "What these parents don't understand is that it may hurt me to know, but that doesn't matter a whit. To us, it's a fundamental matter of right."[9]

Those who favor telling their children they were conceived with the assistance of a donor, along with single mothers or lesbian couples using donor sperm and single fathers or gay men using donor eggs, may wrestle with the issue of donor anonymity. Should a child know the donor's identity? Some parents of donor-conceived children are also concerned about their children's right and ability to locate siblings. Many donors in the United States have donated anonymously, guaranteed by the fertility clinic or sperm bank at the time that their identities would not be divulged. Many parents, similarly, viewing the transaction as akin to donating or receiving blood, intentionally choose anonymous donors. Jenny and Duke, an American couple, opted to go to Spain for IVF with an egg donor, motivated in part by their appreciation of the Spanish approach: all donations are closed (anonymous); compensation to donors is lower, which they felt made it feel less commercialized; and the clinics chose the donor for them, which they viewed as a relief.

Yet advocates of open donation and access to information, such as Wendy Kramer, founding director of the Donor Sibling Registry (DSR), believe that donor-conceived children have a right to know of their genetic origins, not only to know their medical histories but also because "having a complete sense of one's biological origins fosters a more whole identity."[10] In the absence of a national repository of information, Wendy Kramer and her (donor-conceived) son, Ryan Kramer, founded the DSR to help donor families find one another. Begun as a small, private group, the DSR has grown into an organization with global reach. While the number of parents who choose not to register still outweighs those who do so, as of October 2017, the DSR had 55,783 members and had helped to connect more than 14,744 offspring with their half siblings and/or donors.[11]

The DSR has also shed light on the large size of some sibling groups, raising additional worries. With groups of half siblings totaling as many as 150 or 200, there is sufficient concern about the likelihood of donor-conceived children accidentally encountering genetic half siblings that some parents in the San Francisco Bay Area are asking their teenagers to memorize their donor numbers to avoid unknowingly dating a half sibling. Donors too have qualms about the numbers of offspring. One donor, who was promised that his donation would result in low numbers of children, was shocked to learn from the DSR that he has sired seventy children. He now tracks them on an Excel spreadsheet.[12]

Is donor identity a question of privacy or secrecy? Whose rights are paramount? Those of donors who may wish, and in many cases were contractually guaranteed, to be anonymous, or those of the offspring, who may desire to know the identity, or medical history, of their biological parents? Does society have a valid interest in the outcome?

Parents of donor-conceived children are forced to confront these kinds of difficult moral quandaries from day one.

Selecting Sperm

When Claire and her partner, Daphne, decided to have a baby, they knew that their first step would be selecting a sperm bank. Comfortable with the idea of a donor, they were decidedly less at ease with what they quickly came to view as the problematic market for sperm.

They began with their fertility clinic, which was essentially chosen for them as it was the only clinic that Claire's insurance would cover. Meeting first with the director of the well-known clinic's in-house sperm bank, Claire and Daphne were shocked to learn that all donations were anonymous, and that the information available about the donors was limited to only one line of statistics. When Claire asked if it was possible for them to get more information in order to have a more complete profile of the potential father of their child, the director replied that that was neither possible, nor necessary: "I met them, and if I didn't like them, I wouldn't use their sperm." Dejected and certain that this sperm supplier was not a good fit, Claire and Daphne discovered that they could obtain sperm elsewhere and still use it at their insurance-mandated clinic.

The market for sperm has evolved to the point that it is nearly unrecognizable from its origin, more than a century ago. In 1790, the first successful pregnancy by artificial insemination was performed under the care of renegade Scottish surgeon Dr. John Hunter, who advised an infertile couple to have the husband collect his sperm into a warm syringe and then inject it into his wife. More than ninety years later, Dr. William Pancoast, a little-known doctor in Philadelphia, helped a similarly childless married couple conceive by performing the first known successful insemination by sperm donor—unbeknownst to the wife, who had been chloroformed while Dr. Pancoast solicited the donation of sperm from his most handsome student.[13]

From its somewhat dubious inception in 1884 up to the 1970s, sperm donation was performed locally, using fresh sperm, for heterosexual married couples. By the 1970s, the ability to freeze sperm led to commercialization and the birth of the modern sperm bank, which was available only to married couples. The AIDS crisis in the 1980s, which pushed the banks to freeze all sperm in order to test donors for HIV, fueled the growth and scalability of the banks. By 1995, sperm had become a big business, with sperm banks in all fifty states as well as dozens of other countries capable of shipping sperm in liquid nitrogen tanks to any destination. Sperm, in fact, grew to be one of Denmark's top exports.[14] Business exploded over the next twenty-odd years as societal trends turned in its favor, with couples marrying later, or not at all; gay marriage becoming the law of the land; and lesbian couples increasingly pursuing childbirth. In 2017, the typical sperm bank transaction is a far cry from its roots—global as opposed to local, frozen as opposed to fresh, purchased primarily by single women and lesbian couples, rather than their married, heterosexual peers.[15]

Throwing themselves into a nationwide search of this sprawling market, Claire and Daphne discovered that there were two types of donation—anonymous and open—and two types of sperm bank—private and nonprofit. Believing that "the more information the kids have, the better," they knew they were headed for an open donation. As they researched, they learned more about some of the pitfalls of a virtually unregulated market rife with scandals.

In addition to some of the more predictable problems that arise from the lack of limits on numbers of children conceived from a given donor paired with the absence of a system to track these children, there are a host of unexpected challenges arising from what many view as deception and negligence throughout the industry.[16] Clinics have been accused of careless record keeping, mishandling of sperm, and using misleading donor descriptions, and legal cases have been filed against sperm banks claiming fraud, negligence, and breach of contract.[17] One woman attempted to use her husband's sperm to conceive a child after his untimely death. To her shock, all six vials of his sperm—which had a 50 percent chance of carrying Marfan syndrome, which killed him—had been given to other clients. A white woman with a white partner, who purchased vials of sperm from a white donor, mistakenly received African-American sperm.[18] A schizophrenic man with a history of psychiatric hospitalizations and an arrest record who passed himself off as a neuroscientist, unverified by the clinic, sired thirty-six offspring.[19] A child conceived with untested donor sperm that had, unbeknownst to the parents, been in storage for twenty years, was born with cystic fibrosis, and there have been hundreds of donor-conceived kids similarly born with genetic defects.[20]

Claire and Daphne turned toward the nonprofit world, which presented only one option in the United States. The Sperm Bank of California, which considers itself an ethical leader in the field, offered them their three most important criteria: a limit of ten families that would receive sperm from the same donor, an identity release program that would enable their child(ren) to access information about their donor if they desired, and a family contact list to facilitate communication with other families with children from the same donor. They also liked that the bank was small, that it tracked all births from a given donor, and that the staff seemed to truly care about their clients. Although the number of active, available donors was fairly limited compared to the larger private sperm banks, Claire and Daphne identified five contenders, for whom they paid for full profiles. After reviewing the medical histories, personal questionnaires, and baby and childhood pictures of the prospects, their choice was clear: a down-to-earth, calm, college-educated, hobbyist athlete with seemingly good social development and a clean medical history.

The difficult part seemingly done, Claire returned to the fertility clinic expecting to proceed with insemination during a natural cycle. The doctor she met with breezily reviewed a medicated protocol with her, despite Claire's protestations that she was not a fertility patient because she had failed to conceive naturally while actively trying; to the contrary, absent sperm, she had never tried to conceive. Much to her surprise, the doctor told her that her blood work indicated that she had a very low chance of getting pregnant. Despite Claire's request to try a natural cycle, and her attempts, based on a scientific article she had read—to question the need for their protocol given her particular circumstance—she was funneled toward the medicated cycle. Instructed by her doctor to choose between oral or subcutaneous medications, feeling isolated, overwhelmed, and fearful of being unable to conceive, Claire reckoned that she had no option but to use the injectable hormones. Although the drugs worked "so well" that she had multiple eggs, the clinic never counseled her on her options, or warned her of the risk of multiples. They proceeded as planned with the insemination.

To their shock, Claire and Daphne learned at her first ultrasound scan that Claire was pregnant with four babies. Already enormous in her first trimester, feeling horrible and afraid, she and Daphne had to sort through their options. Worried about the impact of carrying four babies to term as well as the risks of selective reduction, she asked her clinic for help and support, and to possibly put her in touch with others who had been in her shoes. She was met with silence.

At thirty-three weeks, five days, nearly twenty weeks after a stressful reduction procedure, Claire gave birth to two small but very robust boys. Shortly after their birth, she and Daphne registered them on the family contact list, hoping to find any half siblings. When the twins were four and a half years old, a family with a daughter of the same donor signed up. The families got together when the kids, almost the same age, were nearly six. One of the boys looked exactly like his half sister. The children got on well, and the families plan to keep in touch. Remarking that she didn't know how unusual their experience was, Claire was surprised that more families hadn't joined the sibling registry.

It turns out that experiences like Claire and Daphne's are happening with increasing frequency. Eleven half siblings between the ages of five and twelve from five families met in Orlando for a "family reunion" in 2016.[21] Zoe, who has twenty-eight half siblings, has met half of them—two, quite remarkably, by accident—and has also met her donor. Sarah and Jenna discovered that they have twenty-one half siblings and met several of them, along with their donor, at a gathering in Cape Cod. Susanna, a mother of two belonging to the supersize sibling group now believed to number as many as two hundred half siblings, took a seven-week, six-thousand-mile, twenty-four-state, cross-country trip with her two donor-conceived kids to meet eleven of their half siblings.[22] Will relationships like these give new meaning to the idea of extended family?

The Egg Hunt

Pietro and Peter found the donor selection process to be an uneasy one. As two men, it was, of course, clear to them that they would need an egg donor once they decided to have a child with a surrogate. This simply fast-forwarded them to the awkward stage of selecting their donor.

"To know that you are deliberately choosing the genetic material of
your future child," Pietro mused, "it is not how you expected it would
be. It's like invading someone's life without them knowing it," he told
me, referring to reviewing the detailed profiles of potential donors.
Working with an agency in Houston, he and Peter had far more information available to them than Richard and I had in Moscow: baby, teen,
and adult pictures; health records; family history; academic history;
previous donations; and success rates. "That part of analyzing someone,
with a price tag on it, was very strange for me," he recalled with discomfort. Like me, he found it far more difficult than choosing a surrogate.
He was troubled by the idea of shaping his future offspring based on
specific features, and having to figure out which features mattered to
him. "In the real world, life doesn't work that way . . . you don't pick
friends based on tall/short, brunette/blond."

Pietro and I are not alone in finding egg donor selection surprisingly thought-provoking. "It forces you to think about what really matters, or if it matters at all," said a woman who does not generally like
to talk about the fact that she used a donor. While some place great
importance on finding a donor with particular attributes—hair and
eye color, athletic prowess, Ivy League degrees—others, like Paula,
care almost exclusively about the likelihood of success and having a
healthy baby.

Originally told she would need an egg donor at her very first
consultation with a fertility specialist, Paula was livid that the doctor
wasn't willing to at least give her own eggs a chance. But two years
and two miscarriages later, after working with additional fertility specialists and researching her own situation extensively, she made peace
with the idea of using an egg donor. Absolutely determined to have
a baby, she pored over donor profiles, searching for a woman who
"looked and felt" like her. She found a perfect fit, and although not a

proven donor—meaning she had not successfully donated before—Paula decided to go with her gut instincts. The cycle was deemed a success and Paula became pregnant. She was so thrilled that she didn't care at all that she was carrying another woman's egg. Her baby inside was thriving, as confirmed by blood tests and the all-important ultrasound scan when they saw the pulsing heartbeat. Sadly, by the time of her second ultrasound, at nine weeks, the baby's heart beat no more. Their third miscarriage, with what was supposed to be the foolproof donor egg, hit Derrick hard. Squatting next to Paula in the hospital room, he shouted obscenities at the top of his lungs. This was their backup plan. What next?

It took a year for Paula and Derrick to try again, but try they did, back at her prior clinic. Focused exclusively on success this time, Paula worked with one of their recommended proven donors, who produced nine excellent-looking embryos, far greater than she herself had ever had. They transferred three of the embryos to Paula and froze the remaining six. She became pregnant, but quickly miscarried. As with her previous donor pregnancy, the fetus was completely normal. After further consultations and eventual immunology treatments to tame her natural killer cells, they transferred three more of the donor embryos to Paula. Another pregnancy. Another miscarriage. With only three donor embryos left, mounting bills, and falling spirits, Paula and Derrick transferred their last three embryos into a surrogate in February 2012. Just seven months later, together with the dozen or so medical professionals tasked with keeping their tiny preemies alive, Paula and Derrick welcomed their long-awaited twins into the world, with not a thought as to their genetic origin.

Unlike Paula and Derrick, and many others who turn to egg donation, Megan and Scott didn't have fertility problems. They met, fell in love, and got pregnant very easily, the old-fashioned way. Megan had an incredibly smooth pregnancy and gave birth to a beautiful boy. A few days later, they were shocked to learn that their gorgeous, healthy-looking son had sickle cell anemia, a disease affecting 8 percent of African-Americans, which requires that both parents be carriers. Neither knew that they possessed the recessive gene. The diagnosis rocked their world. Overwhelmed by the lifelong care their son would require, and digesting the fact that they faced a one in four chance that a second child would have the same disease, Megan could not fathom having another child. Scott, on the other hand, couldn't fathom not having another child.

After four years of persuasion, Scott convinced her to try for another baby using IVF with genetic testing to screen out any possibility of sickle cell. After running some tests, their doctor advised them that while, at age thirty-nine, Megan could still conceive, their odds of success would be as much as two to three times greater if they used a donor egg. It was a surprise to Megan to hear that she needed an egg donor, especially since she had conceived so easily the first time. It took her a while to get her head around the concept, as well as the expense, but she ultimately decided that it was far more important to her to have a healthy child than a biological child.

Her decision made, the clinic required her to undergo counseling about raising a child that was not biologically hers (one of only 18 percent to do so),[23] and urged her to consider whether she and Scott planned to tell the (not yet conceived) child—a topic they had at this point not even considered. Counseling done, they moved on to the donor selection, a process Megan found somewhat disconcerting. She had a choice between using the clinic's own donors, about which she could see only very basic information, such as height, weight, eye and hair color, medical history, and a baby picture, or a donor from an egg bank or agency, most of which had extensive information online. Starting with the agency websites, browsing through pictures, biographies, and academic background, Megan developed her own criteria, focusing on the donor's motivations, education, and physical similarity to herself. And then, like me, she reversed course. "I decided it was better not to choose on looks alone," she explained, noting that the websites seem to encourage the tendency to look at the beauty queens. She and Scott opted for a clinic donor, specifying only that they wanted an African-American donor. Their first IVF cycle failed, and the lab, maddeningly, had a technical error that destroyed their frozen embryos. Frustrated but undaunted, they tried again, transferring two fresh embryos to Megan. They both stuck, and she found the pregnancy, while challenging with two, to be bonding. "When you carry them for nine months, you definitely feel like they're yours." She laughed. Megan rarely thinks about the donor eggs, other than to be grateful that they brought their beloved, mischievous twins into their family.

I see a future in which people will not use sex to reproduce.

Dr. Lee Silver

Louise's Legacy

The Business of Baby-making

Fortunately for women like Jessica, Paula, Marcy, and me—as well as countless tenacious others—there has never been a better time to be confronting infertility. Technological advances make the previously impossible possible. Women with damaged fallopian tubes can conceive. Men with low sperm counts can conceive. Cancer patients can conceive. Gay couples can conceive. Egg, sperm, embryos, and now even mitochondria can be borrowed. The bounds are being pushed every day, enabling people to have their little "miracles"—those, at least, who have the means and access. For as we all learned, patients need not only grapple with a complex and evolving medical field, they must also learn to navigate a byzantine financial and regulatory landscape.

The Fertility Industry

Modern-day treatment of infertility in the United States and elsewhere is a multibillion-dollar industry, yet few participants—doctors as well as patients—recognize the extent to which patient care is shaped by this fiscal reality. Apart from the obvious financial connotations of the word, identifying infertility treatment as an "industry," rather than a purely medical practice, has important implications for understanding treatment decisions; yet treating infertility is not strictly a commercial experience either. Unlike with most consumer transactions, no patient intentionally decides to enter the fertility marketplace, and few want to acknowledge being there. In my experience, as well as that of virtually all the women I interviewed, the descent into this new world is gradual and sneaks up from behind. Focused solely on the goal of getting and staying pregnant, those who find themselves in this marketplace rarely realize, at least initially, that the treatment of infertility differs in significant ways from the provision of many other medical services. At the start, most tend to approach it as they would any other health issue—assuming that there is a single "best course" of treatment and that their doctors will take their future health into account above all else before determining any course of action. Yet while many patients seek second opinions regarding surgery and the treatment of serious illnesses, it seems that the multitude of fertility patients, to the contrary, tend to follow the advice of one doctor, at least at first, and if it fails, simply move on to the next.

When, very early in my journey, I was first prescribed Clomid to help me ovulate, like many other women, I simply took it as instructed. Despite unbearable headaches and no visible results, I continued to take it. Because my doctor prescribed it. When my high-priced fertility specialist later told me I needed to turn to IVF, despite the fact that I had conceived naturally three times, I eventually succumbed, suppressing strong reservations, because my doctor told me to. Although my insurance didn't cover a single cent of my treatment—the first strong clue that I was stepping out of the boundaries of pure medicine—I wasn't suspicious of protocol. It never occurred to me that some of the standard fertility protocols in place (for example, Clomid for six months, IUI for three cycles) may have been based in part on commercial interests, liability-protection, or common practice—and that there may have been little scientific evidence to support them.

A patient is better served to approach fertility treatment options from the vantage point of an educated consumer. My own evolution from patient (blindly accepting medical advice from my doctor) to proactive consumer (researching the best practices and highest success rates globally) took many years. It was only after I experienced failure after failure that my attitude changed and I started to take control and gain the knowledge necessary to successfully navigate my own path to motherhood.

Infertility treatment is, at its core, a medical practice. It is regarded as such in most countries of the world. It is practiced by medical doctors, who dispense hormones and prescription drugs, and often perform surgical procedures. In countries with national health services, such as the United Kingdom, Canada, Sweden, Australia, and many others, infertility treatments are generally covered, within limits, by their various national health plans. In numerous other countries, insurance companies are required to cover infertility as a medical condition, *which it is.*

But in the United States, infertility treatment inhabits the gray zone: not entirely medical, and in many aspects commercial. It is dispensed primarily in for-profit clinics, often by doctors with ownership interests in labs, sperm banks, and egg-donation centers, as well as by distinguished university researchers who may also work in stand-alone for-profit centers. Insurance coverage is required to be offered in only fifteen states, and the coverage is often too limited in scope to see a would-be parent through to achieve the desired goal of conceiving a baby.[1] In at least four of those states, insurance companies must cover fertility treatments only for married couples, and even then, only with the use of the husband's sperm.[2] Patients must steer their way through an unregulated and fragmented market in which clinics with potentially high-profit motives and inherent conflicts of interest face enormous pressure to increase their publishable success rates. The question must be asked: What impact is this having on the integrity of the science of fertility and on the women seeking treatment?

Regulation, or Lack Thereof

In 2018 in America, the landscape for combatting infertility is still in some respects the Wild West. Assisted reproductive technology (ART) providers—the fertility clinics, ob-gyns, reproductive endocrinologists, embryologists, and others involved in performing IUI, IVF, and other procedures—are largely unregulated, with far fewer restrictions than most medical practices, making it harder for patients to assess the safety and efficacy of treatments. Shockingly, in stark contrast to the panoply of regulations surrounding abortion, there is in fact *only one specific law* regulating treatment of infertility. The Fertility Clinic Success Rate and Certification Act, a lonely federal statute enacted in 1992 as a result of a Federal Trade Commission (FTC) intervention in reaction to false advertising by a fertility clinic, requires only that clinics practicing assisted reproductive technology inform the Centers for Disease Control and Prevention (CDC) of their success rates.[3]

Of course, certain aspects of the provision of fertility services are regulated by federal laws and agencies charged with broad oversight of general operating standards, but there is no single governing body with the primary mission of overseeing infertility care. The Clinical Laboratory Improvement Act of 1988 (CLIA), for example, which was enacted to regulate the quality of laboratory services, established certain requirements regarding personnel qualifications, validation of tests, and quality-control standards. Implemented by the Centers for Medicare and Medicaid Services, the act also applies to assisted reproductive technologies and prenatal genetic testing. The FDA regulates drugs and devices used in IVF treatments, although it does not regulate the procedures themselves, nor does it oversee operations of fertility clinics. Some states, in addition to requiring medical and laboratory licensing, have adopted laws to govern the practice of gamete (egg, sperm, or embryo) donation and storage, mandating, for example, that facilities maintain acceptable equipment and storage conditions and institute tracking procedures for frozen gametes to ensure identification and minimize potential abuse.

But apart from the general goals of assuring basic quality standards, unlike in the United Kingdom, Spain, Australia, and many other developed countries, *there is no federal or state agency in the United States with the mandate to regulate the trickier aspects of infertility treatment*: how many embryos may be transferred during IVF; how many children may be conceived from a single donor; how old can a donor be; the type of medical information that must be supplied to potential parents; delineation of the rights and responsibilities of surrogates and intended parents, among others. There is a veritable minefield of unregulated issues.

In the face of this Swiss-cheese-style government regulation, the US fertility industry is largely self-regulating. The vast majority of fertility clinics are members of one or both of the two major professional organizations in the field: the American Society for Reproductive Medicine (ASRM) and the Society for Assisted Reproductive Technology (SART). To assure patients that their clinic meets quality standards, most reputable fertility clinics also seek certification from the Joint Commission, an organization made up of individuals from the private medical sector to develop and maintain standards of quality in medical facilities in the United States.

When considering treatment from a particular facility, it is a good idea to check for its accreditation, for while Joint Commission–accredited institutions must maintain strict standards, members of SART and ASRM are bound only by their clinical and ethical guidelines as well as an obligation to report their activities. And alarmingly, a CDC study found that only 20 percent of clinics follow these guide-lines.[4] Although clinicians who violate them may face sanctions such as being kicked out of the professional societies, there are rarely legal consequences, and the errant doctors and clinics may still treat patients. The doctor responsible for "Octomom," for instance, was dismissed in 2009 from the ASRM, which cited "behavior that violated the group's standards," after transferring twelve embryos into the womb of Nadya Suleman, but he was not barred from practice at that time.[5] He eventu-ally lost his California medical license in 2011 after being found guilty of gross negligence in two additional cases.

Deprived of rules that can be relied upon, fertility patients must, to a large degree, take it upon themselves to learn not only which clin-ics and avenues of treatment might bring the most success but also, and perhaps more disturbingly, whether proposed courses of action might lead to troubles down the way. Like me, most patients are not aware of this as they begin their journey down the rabbit hole in search of a baby.

In this area of regulation, a key aspect of fertility treatment, the United States is an outlier.

Most developed countries (and many developing countries as well) have clear and enforced regulations regarding many aspects of fertility treatment, which typically address physical and health considerations for a patient as well as ethical concerns for society at large. For example, most European countries, recognizing the risks of multiple pregnancies, limit, generally to one or two, the number of embryos that may be trans-ferred during an IVF cycle. In contrast, in the United States, there is neither federal nor state regulation of embryo transfers, which can lead to both health problems for a mother, and an undue burden on society. Thus, only in America do we have "Octomom," an unemployed mother of six who, after transferring an unthinkable number of embryos to her womb, gave birth to octuplets. And while this story may play well for daytime TV, its impact on society at large raises moral and ethical dimen-sions that should be more fully explored rather than ignored.

Mirroring the lack of restraint on fertility practices, there are no clear rules on what information about potential risks doctors are required to communicate to patients. While doctors are, or should be, concerned about multiples, many patients (myself included) are indifferent to, or even eager to embrace, the possibility of twins, and most fertility clinics are happy to indulge them.

"Our mission is to make a woman pregnant, with almost a whatever-it-takes attitude," says Dr. Mark Sauer, now a professor of obstetrics, gynecology, and reproductive sciences at the University of California, San Francisco, after serving as chief of the division of reproductive endocrinology at Columbia University Medical Center for twenty-one years.[6] Although transferring higher numbers of embryos may in fact increase the odds of a woman getting pregnant, there is no obligation for clinics to sufficiently caution women about the numerous health risks to both mother and baby when there is a multiple pregnancy.

A woman carrying multiples, including twins, is labeled "high risk" for a reason: she faces a higher risk of high blood pressure, gestational diabetes, preeclampsia, anemia, postpartum hemorrhaging, and miscarriage, while her babies have a heightened threat of cerebral palsy, blindness, retardation, and preterm birth. Preterm births, in turn, place newborns in greater jeopardy of death, neurological disabilities, and a variety of other health challenges causing, on top of everything else, extended stays in hospitals.[7] Extended stays in a hospital present not only an inordinate expense for a family to bear, but also cost the US healthcare system more than $26 billion per year.[8]

Paula and Derrick experienced this firsthand. When they turned to surrogacy after five miscarriages, their surrogate, Amy, carrying twins, went into labor at twenty-six weeks and four days. Their son was born first, their daughter three minutes later, in a breech position and with a brain bleed. The family's three-month neonatal intensive and intermediate care experience began. In addition to repeated blood transfusions for both babies, their daughter underwent heart surgery at two weeks old while their son endured four hernia operations in his first couple of months of life. Both lived on oxygen tanks for months.

Although many women and couples enter fertility clinics with a stated aim of having twins, an understandable goal given the expense and difficulties of IVF, they often have no understanding of these risks, which are largely preventable, and studies have shown that when patients are better informed, their desire for multiples sharply declines.[9] Yet despite the risks to mother and baby, the incidence of twins has risen by more than 75 percent over the last twenty years. In 2017, nearly four in ten children conceived through IVF were twins.[10] While some doctors defend the decision to transfer multiples by claiming that they are giving patients what they want, Dr. George Annas, a bioethicist and director of the Center for Health Law, Ethics & Human Rights at the Boston University School of Public Health, rejects the justification of accommodating patients as a reason for transferring multiple embryos: "(In) no other field of medicine would the excuse for not doing good medicine be 'the patients demand it.' That's ridiculous."[11]

Patients likewise are often not apprised of the risks associated with medicines or specific treatments that are prescribed for them. In my case, when IVF failed repeatedly, several doctors increased my hormone levels. In taking the higher dosages, was I risking ovarian cancer? Cervical cancer? Some unforeseen risk from the immunological suppression I was undergoing? Largely uninformed of potential fetal risks, I never worried about the long-term effects the treatments might have on my embryo, or baby. Unwarned, I never dreamed that the treatments I believed were helping might actually be hurting my own tiny eggs.

It is not only IVF and the number of embryos transferred that goes unregulated in the United States. Procedures involving controlled ovarian stimulation and IUI are likewise unregulated. Relationships with surrogates are unregulated. Sales of sperm, eggs, and embryos are unregulated. The number and location of offspring from donors is not tracked or regulated.

Long-standing industry guidelines regarding egg donor compensation—stating that payment to an egg donor in an amount over $5,000 requires "appropriate justification" and in an amount over $10,000 is "not appropriate"—have been riddled with criticism and are often disregarded.[12] This is particularly troubling, as the $80 million US egg-donation market is exploding, with older moms, gay couples using surrogates, and cancer survivors entering the marketplace like never before, in addition to the ever-increasing number of traditional heterosexual couples facing unexplained infertility. Donor eggs were used in nearly twenty thousand monthly cycles in 2012, compared with fewer than twelve thousand a decade earlier.[13]

The commercial nature of egg and sperm donation is obfuscated somewhat by the terminology that is used. Payments for egg and sperm are a notoriously long-ignored subject in this country, with the women and men providing the genetic material to babies born through ART known as "donors" rather than "sellers," and the payment to them intended to reflect the time and inconvenience—and, for women, potential health risks—involved in the process of obtaining the eggs and sperm, rather than buying the actual eggs and sperm. Yet the compensation guidelines for egg donors—originally keyed off a multiple of sperm donor compensation, to reflect the greater time spent, plus an uptick for the misery of the process—have, since their inception, been perceived by many as an injustice. Harvesting eggs requires injections, ultrasounds, an invasive procedure, and potential health risks, while harvesting sperm requires one trip to a clinic and a few magazines.

In theory, the egg donor guidelines, intended to protect low-income younger women from being lured into donating their eggs for high pay, also aimed to keep the price of fertility low, benefiting intended parents.[14] However, as the clinics that sell the eggs to the intended parents are not similarly regulated, they are left free to reap profits. And to top it all off, it turns out that the guidelines are largely ignored by a clientele that includes future parents who are willing to pay whatever it takes to have their desired children, as well as women who are willing to help out for a sum that they feel adequately compensates them for the pain and the risk.

"The guidelines are a joke," according to Andrew Vorzimer, a lawyer and law professor who specializes in reproductive law. "I've drafted contracts for egg donors in the six figures."[15] Demand for quality egg donors, or egg donors with specific traits, has helped shape a landscape in which certain donor profiles command higher fees: Asians, Jews, and Ivy Leaguers top the charts, and repeat donors can be paid in the range of $40,000 to $50,000 per harvest.[16]

Equally, or perhaps even more concerning, the ceiling imposed by the guidelines has not diminished the practice of "luring," which continues to flourish in ads, on the Internet, and in other arenas. While strolling through a large summer festival recently, complete with the expected Ferris wheel, whirling teacups, cotton candy, and frozen custard, I saw, wedged between the handmade alpaca sweater and bath-bomb booths, a table with free giveaways—lip gloss, nail files, tote bags, pens in cute colors. The promotion? Recruiting egg donors. As is common on college campuses today, young women flocked to spin the prize wheel, receiving, along with their jumbo nail groomer, pamphlets on the benefits—including payment of $6,000—of sharing their sought-after eggs with those in need.

Donors themselves recognize the commercial nature of the industry. In 2011, four named plaintiffs,[17] representing potentially thousands of similarly situated donors, joined together to bring a class action suit against the reproductive technology professional associations (ASRM and SART), their fertility clinic members, and all egg donation agencies that agreed to abide by the ASRM and SART egg donor compensation guidelines, claiming that the compensation guidelines constituted an illegal price-fixing agreement in violation of US antitrust laws.[18] After nearly five years working its way through the court system, the parties reached a settlement agreement in 2016, with the ASRM agreeing to drop the language restricting financial compensation from its egg donor guidelines.[19]

"Our whole system makes no sense," said Debora L. Spar, author of *The Baby Business*, which presents a thorough and thoughtful investigation of the subject. Referring to the "yuck factor of commodifying human eggs," Dr. Spar believes that "we should either say, 'Egg-selling is bad and we forbid it,' as some countries do, or 'Egg-selling is OK, and the horse is out of the barn, but we're going to regulate the market for safety.' "[20]

But we don't. We don't forbid it. And we don't regulate it.

The absence of regulation not only affects pricing in what is essentially a commercial market, it may also leave patients struggling to assess the health risks as well as the odds of success of desired procedures. Is controlled ovarian stimulation the best protocol for a certain patient? Is a patient better served by IVF? How many embryos should be transferred in a given IVF cycle? How much follicle stimulation hormone (FSH) is too much? Is there any link whatsoever between IVF cycles and cancer risk?

It is common practice in many fertility clinics, for example, for patients to undergo a fairly standard progression of treatments on the road toward IVF. First, a woman will undergo treatment using controlled ovarian stimulation, which involves following a hormone protocol designed to encourage the body to produce as many eggs as possible using clomiphene citrate (Clomid), letrozole (Femara), or FSH, in conjunction with trying the old-fashioned way or through IUI. Generally, it is only after six cycles of some type of controlled ovarian stimulation that a patient then moves on to IVF. Research trials, however, have shown that women who followed a fast-track protocol, skipping three cycles of controlled ovarian stimulation and progressing quickly to IVF had *higher* rates of pregnancy and live births and *lower* costs.[21] In other words, in many cases it would make sense for a woman who does not succeed within two or three cycles of mild ovarian stimulation to go straight to IVF, preferably with a single or double embryo transfer to limit the risk of multiples. Unfortunately, there is no requirement for fertility clinics to convey this information to patients, and no central repository of information that makes it easy for them to find it.

Similarly, questions surrounding the safety of fertility drugs and hormones are rarely discussed or examined. While all the drugs and medical devices used in infertility clinics are approved by the FDA, some, such as Lupron, are prescribed as an "off label" use, meaning that it is not approved for the use in question, and some are used in dosages considered unwise in other countries. The linkage between fertility drugs and cancer, rarely whispered in the halls of a fertility clinic, remains unclear. Yet many of the women I interviewed mentioned the low-grade anxiety that provides constant background noise throughout their fertility journey. "You just know those drugs are bad for you," Jessica reflects. "You worry, but you keep going." I know I worried, and my husband worried. But in the absence of concrete evidence, we chose to disregard our niggling concerns, and we forged on.

Scientists have found that women who take Clomid for longer than one year may have an increased risk for developing ovarian tumors, particularly among those who did not get pregnant while on the drug.[22] Research on the possible correlations between fertility drugs and breast cancer is all over the map, with some studies showing an increased rate of breast cancer among women who took fertility drugs, some studies finding no impact, and a third group indicating a lower risk of breast cancer specifically among women who took Clomid, which is in the same drug family as the chemotherapy drug Tamoxifen. For every study that finds a cancerous connection, there is a countervailing one that says there is nothing to worry about. While the research findings at this stage are conflicting and inconclusive, one thing is clear: no one is out there policing this for patients, who are left to themselves to get educated on the latest findings and consider the unknowns before making treatment decisions.

How did it get to be this way?

Before and After Louise Brown

Having children is the most basic of human functions, and there is an unspoken assumption that it is something any woman should be able to do. On average, approximately 360,000 babies are born each day worldwide; that's 15,000 births per hour and 250 babies born in a single minute. So it is easy to comprehend why the more than eight million women in the United States each year who have trouble conceiving or maintaining a pregnancy are not only devastated but are often truly shocked by the news.

When they are shocked and desperate, and often feeling inadequate, prospective mothers typically turn to doctors for assistance. And for decades, doctors, particularly infertility specialists, have been inventively and increasingly successfully helping women conceive. But they have been doing so on a playing field with limited knowledge and without an umpire; a field, as described by Arthur Caplan, founding head of the division of medical ethics at NYU School of Medicine, "characterized by strong antiregulatory sentiment because it evolved as a business, not a research enterprise."[23] To understand this unique situation, we must go back to the beginning.

The healthy birth of Louise Brown on July 25, 1978, in England—on the 104th IVF attempt by Dr. Patrick Steptoe and Dr. Robert Edwards— forever changed the fertility landscape. Her birth came after decades of innovative, yet unsuccessful, procedures—such as attempted surgical cures on the ovaries and cervix, gland transplants, extracting testosterone from bulls' testicles and estrogen from the ovaries of cows.[24] Born more than thirty years after Harvard Medical School professor John Rock fertilized a human egg in a glass tube, Louise, the world's first successful "test tube baby," set off both a medical and media frenzy. For her parents, Lesley and John Brown, who had been trying for nine years to have a baby, and the uncountable number of similarly situated couples facing previously insurmountable infertility, Louise's birth was a modern miracle, a cause for celebration and great hope. For fertility specialists, such as Drs. Steptoe and Edwards, who "conceived" Louise, it was both the culmination of decades' long work and the signaling of greater progress to come.

But for many others, particularly religious leaders and political conservatives, it was a sin, a dangerous and troubling intervention by mankind into the natural world, or God's domain. The Roman Catholic Church, steadfast in its opposition to any form of assisted reproduction, declared that "from a moral point of view, procreation is deprived of its proper perfection when it is not desired as the fruit of the conjugal act, that is to say of the specific act of the spouses' union." Protestants shared this view: "Men ought not to play God before they learn to be men, and after they learn to be men they will not play God."[25]

Faced with a conflicted public, the government in the United Kingdom launched a comprehensive evaluation of the medical and ethical implications of IVF that led, years later, to the regulation of in vitro fertilization, including the freezing and donation of embryos. After nearly a decade of inquiry and debate, the Human Fertilisation and Embryology Authority (HFEA) was eventually established in the United Kingdom in 1991 with the mandate to regulate not only the provision of fertility services to families in need but also the fertility research and policies to be implemented as the science evolved. In other words, the HFEA was tasked with dealing with the medical, ethical, and policy issues surrounding fertility, balancing the needs of individual families with society at large.

The process didn't work as smoothly in the United States. Faced with a similarly conflicted public, as well as a great deal of agitation remaining in the wake of the highly controversial *Roe v. Wade* decision in 1973, five years prior to Louise's birth, no such authority was established— then or since. One possible explanation for this failure is that in addition to the medical and scientific challenges assisted conception presents, there is a complex set of moral and ethical policy challenges that those on both the left and the right have been reticent to tackle.

Fertility "is unregulated because it touches on two 'third-rail' issues," according to Arthur Caplan. "It touches on abortion and also the creation of embryos, which politicians run away from because too many people still disagree about the right to use reproductive technologies."[26]

Prior to Louise's birth, the US government had "temporarily" suspended funding for fetal research in response to the backlash from abortion foes angered by the Supreme Court's decision in *Roe v. Wade*. After Louise's birth, as in the United Kingdom, the US government convened a special commission to advise on IVF. And, as in the United Kingdom, the commission recommended that the ban on spending be lifted and that IVF be regulated by the Department of Health. But the debate over assisted reproduction, like that over abortion, was too fierce, and no politician would touch it. The ban on federal fetal research remained, and the provision of IVF services stayed largely unregulated.

Nevertheless, with or without government participation, Louise had been born, and a new chapter in reproductive technology had begun.

The absence of federal support for crucial fetal research in the United States gave rise to expanded private practice and the birth of the for-profit fertility clinic. Despite a moratorium on federal funding for IVF research and other studies involving early human embryos that remains in place today, IVF research continued and, in fact, blossomed in the private sector, although without the federal oversight or ethical review that is required when research is funded with public dollars. The federal government in effect ensured its lack of involvement in 1996, when Congress passed an amendment banning the use of federal funds in research related to the creation of embryos. President George W. Bush continued this trend in 2001 with his ban on the use of new embryonic stem cell lines in research, limiting federal spending to the sixty stem cell lines created prior to August 9, 2001, only twenty-one of which were viable.[27] In 2009, President Barack Obama lifted the moratorium on the federal funding of embryonic stem cell research, yet the legislation banning federal funding of experimentation on human embryos, enacted more than twenty years ago, continues to block this research.[28]

Against this backdrop, for-profit clinics expanded, and profits there were aplenty. What began in 1978 as a medical breakthrough in England—a nation with a national health service—has evolved into a more than $3.5 billion industry in the United States, representing a fourfold increase over the last twenty-five years. According to Market-data Enterprises, in 2012, the *average* US fertility clinic had revenues estimated at $3.5 million. But while clinics and the provision of treatment continued to grow, largely unfettered by regulation, what was the impact of the lack of federal funding on domestic IVF research? Remarkably, in a survey of more than six thousand studies on the effectiveness of assisted reproductive technologies between 2000 and 2008, approximately 80 percent were conducted outside the United States.[29] Notable advances in reproductive technology have been driven overseas—such as mitochondrial replacement therapy, the creation of a baby using the genetic material of three parents, being performed by a United States–based doctor in Mexico.[30]

In this regulatory vacuum, fertility doctors have been left largely on their own to chart their course through self-regulation, a situation that presents both an opportunity and a challenge for a patient new to the world of infertility trying to understand the complex array of treatment possibilities, outcomes, and risks.

The rapidly evolving science is a boon, a lifesaver, the very reason I have my two children. But a patient must also understand the regulatory climate, or lack thereof, and the financial and other incentives underlying proposed treatments, and adopt the point of view of a consumer, aware of the varying players and motives; the fact that treatments can vary widely between clinics and among countries; that what is "standard" in one place may be prohibited in another; and that success rates—which may influence a clinic's treatment protocols—vary dramatically, as do costs.

Obtaining the "priceless," unfortunately, often comes with a steep price.

You can't buy love, but you can pay heavily for it.

Henny Youngman

12

Pricing the "Priceless"

Big Money and the Finance of Fertility

*J*essica, who has been through an uncountable number of hormone shots, egg collections, embryo transfers, and all things fertility related, likes to say that "infertility is not for the weak." Well, in the United States, it is also, unfortunately, not for the poor. The assisted, scientific pathway to parenthood is an expensive proposition. The fertility services industry in the United States is expected to break $4 billion in 2018, with the cost of infertility drugs alone exceeding $500 million.[1] The global market for fertility drugs is expected to reach $4.8 billion in 2017 and analysts anticipate that the global fertility services market will exceed $21 billion by 2020.[2]

Although the average cost of one cycle of in vitro fertilization in the United States is popularly reported as costing approximately $12,400 per cycle,[3] a recent national survey found the actual cost now exceeds

$23,000[4]—a figure consistent with those I spoke with who reported spending between $18,000 and $30,000 per cycle, often coming after several attempts at IUI, costing a few thousand dollars each. Add onto that potential additional costs for drugs ($3,500 to $6,000), genetic testing ($3,000 to $7,000), intracytoplasmic sperm injection (ICSI) ($1,000 to $3,000), egg or sperm donation, or a surrogate. The average patient trying to conceive cycles two to three times—and many, of course, attempt more—bringing the average spend to over $50,000.[5]

Costs for egg, sperm, or embryo donation, or for those who need a surrogate, are, of course, much higher. While donor sperm typically costs in the range of $1,000 to $5,000, egg donation expenses can run from $20,000 to well over $100,000, including agency and legal fees. (Embryo donation, in contrast, averages a comparably lower $7,500 to $19,500 per cycle, as it involves a frozen embryo transfer rather than a full IVF cycle.) A surrogate pregnancy done through an agency can easily top $100,000, and the average cost for a couple to have a child through surrogacy with an egg donor is $75,000 to $200,000.[6]

In assessing the real cost of IVF to patients, researchers from the University of California, San Francisco found that the average cost of *successful* IVF treatment was $61,377, significantly higher than the median cost per IVF cycle of $24,373. Similarly, the cost of successful IVF with donor eggs was $72,642, as compared to the more commonly cited average of $38,015.[7]

There is no way around it: fertility treatment, particularly involving third-party parenting, is expensive, placing it out of reach for many in need. It is also variable, and would-be parents' prospects may be dependent on the vagaries of where they live. Robert and Jeffrey, for example, used an agency, a lawyer, a paid surrogate, a paid egg donor, and a well-respected IVF clinic to facilitate the birth of their daughter. Despite a price tag of more than $200,000, they were extremely happy. Happy enough, in fact, to go for a second child using the same agency, egg donor, and surrogate—this time resulting in identical twin boys, a relative bargain at a total cost of $150,000.

Rebecca and her husband, however, were not as fortunate. Despite combined medical, legal, and agency fees of more than $100,000, their surrogacy attempts via repeated IVF cycles failed to deliver the child they hoped for.

Across the pond in London, Alice, a cancer survivor who could no longer carry a baby, sought to have a baby with a surrogate using her own eggs (removed before her chemotherapy) with her husband's sperm. Although the free round of IVF often provided by the British National Health Service was not available to the surrogate, their total medical costs were approximately $6,000, substantially lower than in the United States. There were no legal fees, and as surrogacy in the United Kingdom is legally uncompensated apart from reimbursement of expenses, their total compensation to their surrogate was about $15,000, rendering their total out-of-pocket expenses to have their baby in the region of $21,000—certainly not a small amount but a fraction of the cost to many in the United States.

And Jenny and her husband, Duke, learning that they needed an egg donor after a year and a half of failed fertility attempts and mounting expenses at home in the United States, traveled to Barcelona in hopes of more cost-effective treatment in a medical environment that appealed to them. Less than the price of six eggs at their clinic in the United States, their total treatment costs in Spain amounted to 10,000 euros: 7,500 euros for the IVF cycle, including the donor; 1,500 euros for medicine for the donor; and 1,000 euros for medicine for Jenny. Jenny and Duke were well rewarded for their efforts. Their donor produced eight eggs, seven of which were viable, and Jenny gave birth nearly nine months later to a beautiful, healthy baby girl.

Paying for IVF: The Fertility Casino

Unfortunately, there is not much help available in the United States for would-be parents facing the steep costs of fertility. Fewer than a third of states require insurers to offer coverage for infertility diagnosis and treatment,[8] and among those that do mandate some form of insurance, many exclude IVF treatment altogether, limit the number of cycles covered per patient to as few as one, do not require coverage by employers who self-insure, or cap the monetary benefits to amounts as low as $15,000. These restrictions mean that relatively few women or couples have insurance benefits that can see them through the long haul of taking home a baby. In fact, in contrast with many other costly medical treatments that are covered by health insurance, approximately 85 percent of infertility treatment expenses are paid for out of pocket.[9]

Faced with expensive treatment and inadequate insurance, patients are increasingly turning toward other funding options. Loans in some form—ranging from specialized fertility loans[10] and personal loans to funds provided by lending clubs and home equity lines of credit—are the predominant option; a 2015 survey conducted revealed that 70 percent of respondents incurred debt from fertility treatments.[11] Families that can't qualify for personal loans may turn to credit cards, which often carry steeper interest rates, and quickly accumulate debt.

In an effort to be more attractive in a fiercely contested marketplace, some clinics now develop competitive pricing plans and "money-back guarantees." Hoping to save money over time, patients are increasingly turning to an array of package plans, offered by an ever-growing number of US clinics (often through financing partners), some of which offer better pricing for essentially buying in bulk, while others, often called baby-or-your-money-back plans, offer refunds. But do these programs actually benefit their participants?

A plain bundled IVF package typically offers a discount for a certain number of cycles paid for in advance, with no refund available. Whether a patient succeeds on the first try, or never succeeds, the clinic keeps the cash. Success, it is important to note, does not necessarily mean the birth of a baby. Frustratingly, some clinics define success as a positive pregnancy test, or making it through the first trimester, rather than a live birth.

In a refund plan, on the other hand, a couple pays a fixed fee, for example $50,000, for the right to go through as many IVF cycles as are needed to produce a live baby. In some programs, such as the multi-cycle refund programs offered by Attain IVF, part of a national net-work of fertility providers that perform more than 25 percent of all IVF procedures in the United States, clients are entitled to receive partial or full refunds based on the specific program they enter. Attain IVF's Two-Cycle Program, for example, offers a potential refund of 50 per-cent of IVF costs to an eligible client that does not have a baby after two retrievals and transfers, while the Three-Cycle Refund Program offers a full refund to an eligible client who is not successful after three cy-cles.[12] In contrast, under the terms of the ARC Success Program—the refund plan offered by Advanced Reproductive Care (ARC Fertility), the nation's largest network of partner fertility clinics—if a patient gets pregnant from her first or second IVF cycle, she is entitled to a refund with respect to money paid for additional cycles, but there is no refund forthcoming if she is never successful.[13] Each program is a gamble, but are you betting for yourself, or against yourself?

Perhaps not surprisingly, skeptics argue that much like casinos, the house always wins. In the fertility version, stacking the deck can mean choosing patients with the greatest chance of success—for example, those who are under thirty-seven, have never had a miscarriage or failed IVF cycle, and have encouraging blood test results. The data, albeit lim-ited in scale, seems to back this up. In a small survey of those enrolled in a baby-or-your-money-back program, 67 percent were successful in their first cycle, far exceeding the national average, and 80 percent were successful after two cycles. (It is notable that 87 percent of these women had two or more embryos implanted, also exceeding the na-tional average.)[14] Ironically, it is precisely those patients who are offered a refund program that likely do not stand to benefit from it. It's like paying a rental car company for insurance when the credit card used to pay for the car already provides sufficient coverage.

While a refund plan would clearly seem more desirable than its non-refundable bundled sibling, due to the generally stringent requirements, not all would-be IVF candidates qualify. Attain IVF's refund packages, for example, consider age, body mass index, and medical history, excluding women over thirty-eight and those with diminished ovarian reserve. The plain bundled packages do not tend to be as strict on who can participate, although success rates of 42 percent on the first cycle and 62 percent after two cycles,[15] again exceeding the national averages, imply that women in these programs are also likely to have better-than-average odds of success, and may in fact not need the program.

Also, although both types of package plans claim to have fixed prices for the bundle, it is critical to understand that the real out-of-pocket cost of treatment may be up to 50 percent greater than the list prices, as the costs of real-world necessities such as diagnostic tests and medication, as well as options such as ICSI, are not usually included in the package prices.

Following in the footsteps of many US clinics, Manchester Fertility launched the first multi-cycle refund plan in the United Kingdom (and perhaps the first outside the United States) in 2014.[16] Administered in partnership with Access Fertility, the program offers to repay up to 70 percent of treatment costs to qualifying patients who failed to have a baby after three IVF cycles. By 2017, Access Fertility offered a range of multi-cycle refund and loan programs in partnership with thirty clinics across Britain.[17]

Acknowledging the Las Vegas–style fertility culture in the United States and the desperation of many trying for a child, Dr. John Zhang of New Hope Fertility Center in New York moved further into the realm of gambling, offering a lottery to give away thirty IVF cycles—representing approximately $1 million worth of treatment—at no cost. In return for this "free" treatment, lottery entrants must forfeit their anonymity, agreeing to be announced on Facebook Live, and commit to foot the bill for the medications. They must also, arguably, prepare themselves for another potential downward spin on the fertility roller coaster, in the event their hopes of winning the lottery are dashed. In introducing the lottery, Dr. Zhang hopes to not only help couples in need but to raise awareness of infertility and the vast size of the community struggling with it.[18]

Profits, Conflicts, and the Impact on Care

Of course, there are reasons that treatment of infertility is more expensive than other fields and more expensive in the United States than in other countries. As Dr. Batzofin points out, doctors in the United States have to pay "incredible premiums for malpractice insurance," and equipping and running a state-of-the-art lab is an extremely expensive endeavor. A sophisticated lab includes "incredibly high-cost equipment—one piece of equipment can cost over $100,000; one ultrasound machine can cost over $50,000." Plus the lab is staffed by highly educated embryologists who must be well compensated. "Is it any wonder that the costs of providing these services are not cheap?" Dr. Batzofin muses. Not to mention the inordinately high prices of the medications in the United States, which can be more than double the cost of the same drugs overseas.

Tellingly, fertility clinics are viewed as a commercial industry even among those who run them. They are in the business of producing embryos and getting women pregnant. Although it is a very special business—the business of helping would-be parents have children, some worry about the implications of it being "a business no different than others."[19] Concerned that business influences, such as the desire for profits, may lead to ethical lapses, Dr. Alan DeCherney, head of the reproductive endocrinology and gynecology affinity group of the Eunice Kennedy Shriver National Institute of Child Health and Human Development (NICHD), noted scandals have become so prevalent that one "can't go through a week without reading something in the paper about reproductive technology." Contrasting this with other medical specialties, Dr. DeCherney, who served as past president of both ASRM and SART and former editor in chief of the medical journal *Fertility and Sterility*, did not "remember a scandal about the treatment of heart disease."[20] Dr. Merle Berger, the founder of Boston IVF and a highly regarded professor at Harvard Medical School, describes his job in distinctly commercial terms: "I manufacture embryos."[21]

Fertility clinics advertise in magazines, on the Internet, on radio, and on billboards. They hire marketing consultants and public relations firms. They cultivate relationships with referring physicians. "We wine and dine them," reports one lab director, "and tell them how good we are."[22] And their efforts are often rewarded. Fertility specialists, such as reproductive endocrinologists, earn almost 50 percent more in salary than general endocrinologists, not to mention the potential profits from entrepreneurial ventures such as egg and sperm donation and lab work.[23]

Fertility treatment is expensive *and* profitable. What impact does the profit incentive have on a patient who walks through the door of a clinic? Or who has already experienced five failed IVF cycles?

Three spin-off effects of the commercial nature of the industry that are particularly worrisome are the innate conflicts of interest, the fragmented nature of the provision of fertility services, and the overemphasis on success rates, all of which can have a significant influence on treatment.

Fertility clinics have a clear profit motive in a market that offers what, for many, is a priceless product, with consumption limited only by a patient's ability to pay. And because many fertility doctors own their own practices (and often the labs, donation agencies, and other ancillary organizations), there is inherent potential for conflicts of interest between their pure practice of medicine and their commercial incentives; that is, what is in the doctor's best interest is not necessarily in the patient's.

Patients who start down the path of fertility treatments describe it as being stuck on a treadmill that they cannot get off; as feeling like they've fallen down a rabbit hole and can't get out; as an addiction, as potent as cigarettes or alcohol. They just can't stop trying. I know I felt that way. As did Paula, and Jessica, and almost every woman with whom I spoke, particularly those who repeatedly miscarried.

When I first met Marcy and listened to her calmly tell me her harrowing tale, she shared with me that she felt that nothing could really help her recover from the loss of her baby other than getting pregnant again. Her confession brought me back over a decade, to my gleaming office in the City of London, where I sat frozen in front of my computer screen, reading a column by the journalist Dahlia Lithwick about her miscarriage. She wrote that she had been warned by a colleague that one never truly recovers from a miscarriage until she gets pregnant again. Now newly pregnant, Dahlia agreed that at least in her case, her colleague was right. Terror struck my heart. I was eighteen months into trying desperately to conceive after my second miscarriage, and I was still not OK. What if I never got pregnant? Would I ever be OK again?

Women who miscarry often think that it might be easier to quit if they had never gotten pregnant. But those who fail to conceive do not tend to agree, especially when there is no explanation for the failures. With no reason to believe that an eventual pregnancy won't stick, and conditioned to hope that the next cycle will work, most find it nearly impossible to give up trying (unless or until the money runs out, of course).

Yet sadly, the more times a woman attempts IVF without success, the less likely she is to succeed the next time around. As strong as the will is to have a child, it may not make sense to keep going. Confounding the situation, the same doctor charged with providing guidance, which may sensibly include counseling her to stop, often stands to profit from one more cycle. In most other fields of medicine, unless a condition is terminal, there is generally an understood stopping point. If the proposed remedy doesn't cure the ill, patient and doctor often move on. But fertility treatments have no such stopping point. The patient, often desperate for a baby, doesn't want to quit. The doctor may advise her that her odds are low, but, similarly, he has no incentive, or requirement, to urge her to quit. It is not that doctors don't intend to, or don't in fact "do the right thing"—of course many do, as in my own case—but unlike most other fields of medicine, the inherent conflict is there. And patients need to understand this innate tension to be able to navigate the waters.

Compounding this tension is the fact that doctors who practice in for-profit clinics, which they may own, often become competitors. The fragmented and competitive nature of the fertility business may impact the evolution of the science as a whole, particularly in light of the dearth of federal funding for research that might yield a greater, and more widely shared, understanding of more of the causes of and treatments for infertility. When a fertility clinic makes a breakthrough enabling its success rates to jump, it gains a competitive advantage, rendering little impetus for the clinic to share its "secret sauce." In contrast to discoveries relating to the treatment of cancer or cardiac problems, for example, where scientific breakthroughs and best practices are shared broadly among practitioners, fertility clinics are incentivized to refine their protocols and tout their greater ability to achieve higher pregnancy rates than their competitors.

Success rates are the metric by which fertility clinics and practitioners live and die, despite the fact that generalized success rates can often be misleading, or worse, manipulated. "Success rates are difficult," says Dr. Sauer, "because everyone looks at a success rate as the baby for which they are trying so hard to achieve. They don't really question the number . . . or ask what that really means to a program. . . . If a program wants to maintain a very high success rate, they can and do literally select the best patients to treat."[24] Clinics also, troublingly, may manipulate their reported success rates, according to Dr. Vitaly Kushnir, a reproductive endocrinologist with the Center for Human Reproduction in New York City who analyzed six years of clinical data reported to the CDC.[25]

Marcy, a fit, healthy marathon runner, confronted this problem. Concerned that Marcy and her husband would have trouble conceiving due to her low ovarian reserve, her ob-gyn referred her immediately to a top fertility clinic, nationally recognized for its success rates. But

Marcy was a challenging case, and she quickly sensed that the doctors at the clinic were not keen to treat her. "I felt like they were saying, 'We don't want to do IVF because you are going to ruin our statistics,' " she recalls bitterly, "especially because I was so young."

The variability of success rates across age groups further muddies the analysis. For example, while 29.2 percent of all fresh (non-donor) IVF cycles in the United States resulted in a live birth in 2013, women under age thirty-five experienced a live birth rate of 39.9 percent, while the odds of a live birth for women over forty-two was only 5.2 percent and for women over forty-four, just 1.6 percent.[26] So a patient studying success rates from clinic to clinic must look very specifically—and realistically—at patients in her age group, particularly those facing similar challenges or using similar protocols. Marcy learned this as well. In searching for a second clinic, she pored over the success-rate charts provided by the clinics as well as what she could find from the CDC, looking furtively for cases that fit her profile. Perhaps not surprisingly, at the renowned clinic that was reluctant to treat her, she found none.

Possibly because people considering IVF are hopeful to have children, research shows that patients facing treatment tend to vastly overestimate their odds of success. Perhaps aspiring parents would more accurately perceive their chances if pregnancy rates were relayed in a form that more clearly conveys the high rates of failure, such as "70.8 percent of all fresh (non-donor) IVF cycles *did not* result in a live birth in 2013."

Yet in the face of a flawed system, patients shop for the clinics with the highest success rates, and clinics do everything in their power to oblige, pumping their rates as high as they can and publishing them. The pressure to keep numbers up forces clinic directors to face extraordinarily difficult choices about whom to treat, knowing that the harder the case, the lower the odds of success, which may hurt the clinic's statistics and the overall image of the program. This intense focus on reporting success rates "actually drives clinics to provide sub-optimal care," according to Dr. Kushnir, who consults part-time with the CDC in an effort to improve the data reporting methodology. "There is motivation to report best outcomes."[27]

Marcy well remembers her shocked response to being told she was not the "right" fit for her chosen clinic: "I am offering you $100,000 to basically do nothing and you still won't treat me?" Acknowledging that some clinics "cherry-pick their patients to artificially inflate their reporting," Dr. Batzofin adds that this is certainly not the case with all clinics, emphasizing that there are clinics, like his, "that treat patients, not numbers."

In addition to determining who gets treated, the heavy emphasis on success rates can also affect the treatment protocol of patients, producing a unique combination of conservative and aggressive medicine. On the conservative side, doctors often prefer to stick to protocols that have worked for others in the past; many are understandably cautious when considering innovative treatment, wanting to minimize the risk of a patient not conceiving a baby, or of harming their own publishable statistics.

On the aggressive side, some clinics will take the "kitchen sink" approach, trying anything and everything that has worked before, often prescribing protocols and drugs that may not be specifically medically indicated, all in hopes of achieving the desired pregnancy. Notably, Lord Robert Winston, an eminent British fertility researcher and clinician who now serves as professor of science and society and emeritus professor of fertility studies at Imperial College London, concerned about the proliferation of fertility treatments in the United Kingdom (a country with far greater regulation than the United States) warned fellow academics that "we have gotten carried away with massive enthusiasms in reproduction. That mixture of enthusiasm and patient desperation is actually a very toxic and heady mixture. It is worthwhile standing back a little from the technologies that we employ."[28]

The paramount importance of success may also lead some clinics to push for strategies with a higher likelihood of a pregnancy, despite a patient's wishes. Paula, for example, who switched clinics a few times, felt pressure at her first clinic to go straight to an egg donor for her very first cycle, despite her strong desire to try with her own eggs. Marcy felt the same pressure. "Do they make more money when they use donor eggs?" she asked me, puzzling over the fact that so many women she knows were urged in this direction, even before trying one cycle of IVF with their own eggs. (In some cases, they do.)

Sometimes the quest for success leads fertility clinics in the United States to transfer more embryos than may be beneficial or desirable for a healthy pregnancy. In the case of "too much" success, parents of potential multiples must face the often painful and heartbreaking decision to either continue with a likely challenging pregnancy and childbirth, or to selectively reduce. After five years of trying to have a baby, Paula and Derrick faced the hardest decision of their lives when told that their surrogate was pregnant with four babies, and if they did not terminate the pregnancy of two of them, there was a very high risk of the surrogate miscarrying all four of them. To this day, Paula can't speak of it without crying, remembering the agony of that decision, especially after she and her husband had been struggling so long to create life.

But it doesn't need to be this way.

A New Measure of Success?

The drive to transfer multiple embryos hinges to a great extent on the definition of "success," which is calculated for the all-important CDC success-rates table as the number of pregnancies achieved *per cycle*. One cycle of IVF is defined in America as a cycle in which freshly generated embryos or previously frozen embryos are transferred to the womb. This means that if a woman who has a successful egg harvest elects to transfer only one healthy-looking fresh embryo (while freezing the rest) and does not become pregnant, then opts to transfer a second (frozen) embryo from the original retrieval in a subsequent cycle and does conceive, the clinic will have produced one failure followed by one success.

If the same clinic had transferred two embryos to the same woman during the first transfer cycle, and the woman conceives one of them, the
clinic would be credited with one success and no failures. So the clinic
is clearly motivated to transfer more embryos to increase the odds of
success the first time.

But while the CDC method for measuring success may make sense
in the statistical world, it doesn't necessarily make sense in the real
world. There is an ever-growing body of evidence indicating not only
that elective single embryo transfers (eSETS) are safer for a woman
undergoing IVF, avoiding the risk of multiples, but also, significantly,
that clinics do not experience declines in their success rates when
transferring single embryos. In Sweden, Belgium, and parts of Canada,
where eSET is on the rise as a result of both regulation and encourage-
ment through strong financial incentives, multiple births have been dramatically reduced while live birth rates have been maintained.[29]

So what is holding clinics and patients back from more single embryo transfer in the United States? The expense of each IVF cycle, the
lack of insurance coverage for the majority of the country, and the way
success rates are calculated and presented.[30]

Expanding insurance coverage would clearly help to alleviate the
current climate in which patients are driven or even forced by financial
circumstances to try to maximize their pregnancy odds each cycle by
transferring multiple embryos, despite health risks and potential long-
term costs. Higher coverage limits or providing benefits for more cycles
would also restore the ability of patients to make decisions that are in
their own or their families' best interests. While it may seem that an
expansion may be too costly to impose on employers or the public,
evidence points to the contrary: more than 90 percent of employers
that included infertility coverage in their company health insurance reported that the increased coverage did not have a measurable, significant increase in the cost of their plans.[31]

Citing the moral hazard created by the toxic combination of expensive treatment and inadequate health insurance, a group of fertility

specialists at the Hastings Center and Yale Fertility Center persuasively suggest that a simple change in calculation of success rates would help patients, both in terms of their treatment, and, for those lucky enough to have insurance, in the way their insurance benefits are calculated. In their view, a "cycle" should include the transfer of all embryos generated during one egg collection cycle. That is, one cycle would include a complete series of events: the egg collection and initial fresh embryo transfer, if any, followed by successive frozen embryo transfers until either a pregnancy is achieved or all the embryos from the original collection have been transferred.[32] This approach would more accurately reflect the results of the eggs collected per harvest—particularly in cases of egg freezing and freezing of embryos undergoing genetic screening, both of which result in no transfer at the time of collection—and would achieve good pregnancy rates without multiple births. Perhaps most important, it would diffuse the unrelenting pressure to try to get a woman pregnant in a given cycle at all costs.

"Fertility Tourism"

The search for the intersection of a high quality clinic, a jurisdiction with favorable laws, and—a deal breaker for many—a price point that is manageable, leads many to travel to wherever it is on earth that they can find, and afford, what they need to have a baby. Traditionally thought of as traveling abroad to receive treatment in a different country, fertility tourism for Americans is often domestic as well as international, with New Yorkers traveling to California and Michiganders hopping over to Illinois.

While the United States, with its limited regulation, is often a destination for Europeans from countries like Germany and Italy with more restrictive laws, US fertility seekers turn to countries like Israel, India, Spain, and Mexico for IVF, particularly with donor eggs, because of their high success rates and lower costs.[33] Russia and Ukraine have been gaining popularity as well over the last decade, due to the cost-effective success (approximately $3,000 in Russia and $1,800 in Ukraine for a single cycle of IVF) in a climate with favorable laws, including with respect to surrogacy and donation.[34] Experts estimate that the Russian IVF market, which reached nearly $400 million in 2015, will grow to $641 million by 2022, fueled in large part by its low costs in combination with advanced IVF facilities and treatment options.[35]

It is not only those needing a third party who travel. Some would-be parents, for example, pick a jurisdiction where they can choose the gender of their child. As many as one in five couples who seek treatment at HRC Fertility, a network of clinics in Southern California, go for "family balancing," or nonmedical sex selection.[36] While growing in popularity, family balancing is controversial, with global agencies such as the United Nations and World Health Organization opposing sex selection for nonmedical reasons. Banned in numerous countries, including Australia, Canada, China, India, and the United Kingdom, gender selection performed using preimplantation genetic diagnosis (PGD) is currently legal in the United States, Mexico, Thailand, and a handful of other nations, although clinics have their own rules about using the technology in the absence of a medical need.

Traveling in search of a baby has become so common that it has spawned its own name, "fertility tourism" or "reproductive tourism," and a host of books and movies. *Google Baby*, an Israeli documentary, tracks gay Israeli men who set off on a journey to purchase eggs in the United States and procure a gestational surrogate in India, resulting in the birth of an Israeli-American baby on Indian soil. The book *Cosmopolitan Conceptions: IVF Sojourns in Global Dubai*, by Yale professor Marcia Inhorn, tells the stories of twenty-one couples based on interviews with "reprotravelers" from more than fifty countries seeking treatment at one fertility clinic in Dubai; these seekers hail from other nations in the Middle East where IVF is not allowed; from the east coast of Africa where it is not available; from Europe to bypass laws; from Australia, South Asia, and even a few from America, primarily to save on costs. Ironically, living and working in Dubai, I went to Russia for treatment.

When people can't get what they need in one country, they will go to another, if they have the means.

Making life even more complicated for "reprotravelers"—a term I much prefer to fertility tourist, as I certainly never thought of myself as a tourist in my laser-focused medical excursions—is the fact that even in the overwhelmingly joyous event that they hit the jackpot and have their much anticipated, much desired baby, if the family worked with a donor or surrogate, the challenges to becoming a parent don't necessarily stop at birth. Much as there is no standard protocol in the provision of ART, chaos reigns with regard to the legal status of cross-border babies.

Enid is a single mother with dual Israeli and American citizenship.[37] While living in New York, she conceived her first child with the use of a sperm donor arranged by her New York fertility clinic. When she went back to the same clinic in hopes of giving her son a baby sibling, she unexpectedly ran into egg-quality concerns she did not experience the first time. She turned to a donor egg, using sperm from the same man who sired her son, so that her son and his little brother or sister would be genetically related. Happily, the IVF worked. While pregnant, Enid and her son moved back to Israel, where her daughter was soon born.

When a baby is born to a US citizen overseas, the child's parent or parents must contact the nearest US embassy to apply for a consular re-port of birth abroad of a citizen of the United States of America (CRBA) to document that the child is a US citizen. The CRBA is critically impor-tant. It is proof of citizenship, and is necessary to obtain a US passport. In a bizarre catch-22, because a baby born to a US citizen is deemed to acquire US citizenship at birth, and because no US citizen can enter the United States with any passport other than a US passport, the newborn cannot enter the United States without a US passport, even if he or she has a valid foreign passport—even if the United States has declined to grant the family a CRBA. Without the CRBA, therefore, an American parent cannot legally bring his or her baby "home."

When Enid went to the US embassy in Israel to register her daughter, she naturally told them that she was a single mother, a fact made somewhat obvious by the absence of information in the "father" section of the form. When asked about the paternity of her child, Enid willingly divulged that she had used donor sperm. The officer then asked her, quite directly, if she had used a donor egg, to which she gave her shocked assent. Enid was summarily informed that she could not transfer her citizenship to her daughter, as citizenship is transferred only through DNA (although this is clearly not the case with adoptive parents). She needed proof that one of the donors was a US citizen. Both the egg and sperm donations were made in New York, most likely by US citizens, but her donors were anonymous, and there was no way to prove citizenship. Despite giving birth to her daughter, breastfeeding her, and having full legal responsibility for her well-being, Enid was told that she could not pass on her citizenship to her.

Fortunately for Enid, and others in her situation, the long-established State Department interpretation of the Immigration and Nationality Act requiring citizens to have a genetic connection to their child was relaxed slightly in 2014, allowing gestational mothers (those who carried their babies) to pass on US citizenship to their children, provided that the gestational mother is considered the child's legal mother under the laws of the birth country. While this is a boon to single mothers like Enid, or to women who may have a same-sex or non-US-citizen spouse or partner, it still leaves many families out in the cold. What about a couple made up of a father who is a US citizen and a mother who is not, who needs to rely on a sperm donor? Or a couple in which the mother is a US citizen and the father is not, which needs to use a traditional surrogate or egg donor and surrogate? Or a binational lesbian couple where the woman who carries is not the US citizen? In each of these cases, since the US citizen, while a legal (and *actual*) parent, did not supply the genes, his or her child is out of luck.

As a lawyer who practiced overseas for nearly a decade, I am no stranger to the vagaries of international law. I had also extensively researched the pros and cons of pursuing fertility treatment in several jurisdictions. Yet when Richard and I decided on the unusual path of transferring embryos to me created of both my own egg and a donor's egg at the same time, *we did not think for one second about any implications for the citizenship of our child.* In our case, had it worked, we theoretically shouldn't have had a problem as we were married and Richard was the genetic father, but it certainly had the potential to make our lives more difficult. When we contemplated using a donor egg with Catherine, our surrogate, had I not had good eggs, we similarly never thought about the citizenship question, and we could have been walking into a minefield.

As it was, as two married US-citizen parents, it was still quite a time-consuming and hair-pulling ordeal extracting our CRBA for our son, William, from the US embassy in London. Although recognized as his mother under English law, and possessing a birth certificate with my name listed as "mother" and Richard's as "father," the embassy official in London had a list of maddening demands. He asked for the hospital records of William's birth, which, of course, listed Catherine as the ad-mitted patient, and asked for our marriage certificate. Again, despite my name on the birth certificate, medical records of my IVF treatment, and a letter from Dr. Oxana providing assurance that the embryos were mine, he classified our son as a child born out of wedlock to a US citizen father and a British mother, a situation that would require Richard to prove paternity, further slowing down the process and adding expense. But the issue to me was much bigger than obtaining citizenship; it was being recognized as my son's legal mother, something that came quite naturally to the Brits.

Frustrated and unable to budge the embassy ourselves, I called Ann, the English court-appointed social worker assigned to guide us through our case. We had known Ann since our daughter, Alexandra, was born, and she had helpfully and cheerfully steered us through the compar-atively straightforward UK process to obtain our parental order and birth certificate. She was as outraged as I was, noting that the US stance of disregarding our British birth certificate was a treaty violation, and she contacted an English judge to ask him to intervene on our behalf. A few days later, we were back at the embassy in front of a Homeland Security officer, now willing to accept my maternity. Finally, after nearly two months stranded in London, we received from the US embassy William's consular report of birth abroad, listing me as his mother and Richard as his father.

Two days later, US passports in hand, our internationally conceived British-American family of four boarded the plane home to New York.

The world is full of hopeful analogies and
handsome dubious eggs called possibilities.

George Eliot, *Middlemarch*

13

The Good, the Bad, and the Eggs
The Fundamental Debate About Egg Integrity

I'd like to believe that I knew at the time how lucky I was to have met Dr. Oxana when I did. But if I didn't know it then, I certainly had figured it out by the time she found good eggs in me. And I was a downright acolyte by the time William was born. But it was when I was sitting quietly in the back of the hotel ballroom in New York City in 2016 observing the ART World Congress that I truly comprehended how fortunate Richard and I were.

I had attended the medical conference as part of my ongoing effort to understand the impact, if any, of IVF on egg quality. Alexandra was nine years old, and William six, and although I was no longer trying to have children, I was still pursuing concrete answers to the questions raised for me that first day I met Dr. Oxana—questions that plagued me during and after my own fertility pursuit and success. I needed to keep digging as part of my effort to help others, but also, honestly, because I couldn't let it go.

In digesting how superior contemporary PGS techniques are to those available when we were trying to conceive, I realized yet again that we had beaten the odds. The ability to test embryos with the remarkable precision that exists in 2017 has shed much light onto the size and nature of the mosaicism problem, which had previously languished in the dark.[1] It turns out that at the time we had our genetic testing for Alexandra, using the first-generation FISH technology, as many as half of the day three embryos tested may have been mosaic. That means that when Richard and I were told in New York in 2006 that three were normal, we were pretty darn lucky that at least one of the two that we transferred actually *was* normal. We had no idea at the time that we were running that risk. We basked confidently in the glow of knowing that we had a perfect little girl growing inside. It also means that when my next two batches of embryos were tested in 2008 using FISH, and none turned out to be normal (zero out of five, followed by zero out of eight), one of those little guys might have turned out all right. But how could we know?

Yet look at what that first-generation technology did for our family: after six miscarriages (many with complex abnormalities) in a row without PGS, we had two healthy children with PGS.

During the 2016 ART World Congress, renowned geneticist and PGS pioneer Dr. Santiago Munné noted that even among those using the most sophisticated PGS techniques, there are stark differences in aneuploidy rates (embryos with abnormal chromosomes) between different fertility clinics and even among doctors within the same clinic. One study, he pointed out, showed the rates of abnormal embryos to range from 18 percent to 60 percent,[2] while the different rates of mosaic embryos ranged from 16 percent to 44 percent.[3] Dr. Munné reflected that these differences likely resulted from the different stimulation protocols and culture media used by the various doctors and clinics. He looked up as he addressed an audience of the world's leaders in the field.

"Aneuploidy is not only produced by maternal age but also by ourselves, by the IVF procedures. . . . We have looked at hormone stimulation forever and it's really hard to pinpoint how this could happen, but it is the likely suspect. We are producing chromosomal abnormalities and we now need to determine how we can improve results just by changing things in the lab."[4]

I sat up straighter in my chair. Was one of the foremost experts in genetic screening in the United States declaring to the scientific community that IVF as commonly practiced here was detrimental to egg quality? That the fertility labs were likely creating some of the chromosomal abnormalities the new technologies were working to weed out?

Dr. Munné concluded his remarks. This could be good news, he said. "If we can create chromosomal abnormalities, we can fix them."

This was music to my ears. Dr. Munné's words lent scientific validity to what I had firmly believed for a number of years. A belief that I felt was so important that it was one of the driving forces that compelled me to write this book.

I looked around me to gauge the reaction of the crowd. In a roomful of scientists, researchers, and practitioners from abroad, far more heads than I expected were nodding in agreement.

I was also very gratified to hear Dr. Munné's words because, while I have long believed that Richard and I would not have our precious children if not for the existence of PGS, I am also well aware that the PGS would not have been worth much if, as I had been told, I indeed had no good eggs, and therefore no good embryos, left to find. Luckily for Richard and me, we had decided to give Dr. Oxana's radical "philosophy" on non-static egg quality a chance. A philosophy that I had just heard legitimized by one of the top fertility scientists in the United States.

All About Eggs

Egg quality, it turns out, not only matters, it is everything. Without a healthy egg, there can be no healthy embryo. What do women with infertility, repeated IVF failures, and multiple miscarriages have in common? Abnormally high numbers of eggs with chromosomal abnormalities.

While most US fertility doctors have traditionally advocated the position that chromosomal errors in eggs accumulate gradually over thirty to forty years and are beyond our control, multiple research studies show that many chromosomal abnormalities actually occur in the couple of months before an egg is ovulated,[5] indicating that improving the quality of eggs is, to some extent, within our control.

As conventional wisdom maintains, girls are born with a set number of eggs. However, the eggs, which begin developing in the tiny ovaries in utero, are not mature, or fully developed at birth; rather, each immature egg exists in a state of suspended animation, waiting its turn to develop into a fully mature egg, capable of surviving ovulation and perhaps fertilization. (The vast majority of eggs, incidentally, will die off in the process.) The eggs grow and develop through a process called meiosis, a complex mechanism of cell division and recombination by which immature eggs create their own distinct genetic patterning—their DNA—as they develop into mature eggs. An egg starts out as a single cell, which divides into two, then divides again into four, each time ejecting copies of chromosomes. Ideally, each of the four daughter cells has a single strand of twenty-three chromosomes, half the chromosomes of the original parent. Sperm similarly go through meiosis, through a slightly different process, and end up with a corresponding string of twenty-three chromosomes. When fertilization occurs between one sperm and one of the four daughter cells, the chromosomes pair, resulting in forty-six chromosomes in the embryo. When something goes wrong in the process, abnormalities—such as a missing chromosome or an extra chromosome—result. These chromosomally abnormal eggs—aneuploid eggs—when fertilized, form aneuploid embryos, the vast majority of which miscarry.

Although meiosis begins and is largely completed while a female fetus is still in the womb, each egg does not go through its final stage of meiosis until many years later, approximately six to sixteen weeks before it is ovulated. There is, therefore, a long time period, lasting throughout a woman's entire reproductive life span, in which things can go awry. Contrary to the long-held view that chromosomal abnormalities occur gradually over decades as a woman ages, numerous European studies clearly indicate that many chromosomal abnormalities in eggs arise during the final stages of meiosis, occurring in the weeks and months before ovulation.[6] What's more, embryos obtained through IVF more frequently have multiple complex abnormalities that occur during this latter stage of meiosis than those of naturally occurring pregnancies, in which abnormalities usually involve only a single error from a far earlier stage of development.[7]

If we know that the environment during meiosis, not merely the passage of time itself, can foster the development of abnormal eggs, we can change the environment.[8] There is a brief window of opportunity during the growth phase before ovulation in which women can increase their odds of developing healthy eggs, through, for example, increasing certain nutrients and supplements known to support normal egg growth and development, and eliminating exposure to known toxins, such as BPA and phthalates.

Understanding this window of opportunity is important for those trying to conceive on their own; and it is critical to anyone undergoing or considering assisted reproductive technologies. For it is precisely during this time of meiosis that women undertaking IVF undergo ovarian stimulation protocols, which—as we now know—at high levels, may have a negative effect on egg quality.

In 2002, distinguished reproductive technology expert Lord Winston, in response to a study that indicated a high number of chromosomally abnormal embryos following IVF, noted that it was "not clear whether the incidence of chromosomal abnormalities is increased after administration of gonadotropin, perhaps as a result of over-riding natural checkpoints."[9] Lord Winston speculated that "the majority of these chromosomal abnormalities may arise after resumption of meiosis, just before ovulation" and remarked that it was worrying that elevated in-cidence of chromosomal abnormalities following IVF "has attracted so little attention from those practising and regulating IVF."[10]

In spite of his prominence, Lord Winston's theory remained largely unexplored for years. Yet over the last decade, research teams in the Netherlands,[11] Spain,[12] Italy,[13] India,[14] Japan,[15] and Russia[16] have found that conventional ovarian stimulation protocols may have a negative ef-fect on egg quality, causing women to produce fewer normal eggs and embryos than those with a mild stimulation protocol (or no stimula-tion at all). In study after study, these scientists concluded that lower doses of stimulation drugs could significantly improve embryo quality and fertilization rates.

This is an exciting time for confronting infertility, for if egg quality is not predetermined and does not follow a one-way street into decline, then women can theoretically—and in reality it turns out—improve their egg quality and increase their chances of conceiving a healthy baby. As the conventional Anglo-American thinking about eggs is being turned on its head, there are both natural and interventional methods available to right the sinking ship.

Optimizing Your Environment for Healthy Eggs

"Widespread exposure to toxic environmental chemicals threatens healthy human reproduction," the International Federation of Gyne-cology and Obstetrics warned in a landmark statement in 2015.[17] The announcement was made largely in response to the rampant growth of endocrine disruptors, chemicals found in many everyday products that imitate sex hormones and often confuse the body's own systems. Endocrine disruptors are everywhere, lurking in items ranging from plastics, food cans, and cash register receipts to personal care products like soaps, shampoos, and cosmetics. The Endocrine Society, an interna-tional association of doctors and scientists specializing in the hormonal system, concurs, noting the mounting evidence linking endocrine disruptors to infertility, as well as a host of cancers (breast, uterine, ovarian, testicular, and prostate, to name a few). We are unwittingly exposed day after day.

Yet pairing awareness of how our environment affects us with a greater understanding of the time frame in which our eggs are maturing and forming their genetic material opens the door to exciting new possibilities. Armed with this knowledge, women can actually improve their chances of developing healthy eggs in as little as two to three months.

Key vitamins such as folate (a B vitamin, or folic acid, its synthetic supplement), B_6, B_{12}, and Coenzyme Q_{10} (CoQ_{10}), for example, have all been shown to play important roles in the development of healthy eggs, the smooth operation of the ovulatory process, and the quality of embryos.[18] Folate, widely recognized for its impact in preventing birth defects, also plays an important function in making new copies of DNA when a cell divides, rendering it essential at every stage of fertility, from egg to fetal development.[19] Multiple studies from a range of countries demonstrate the significance of adequate levels of folate and vitamins B_6 and B_{12} on the development of healthy eggs;[20] a Dutch group found that women with twice as much folate as their peers were three times as likely to conceive in a given cycle, and that women with higher levels of vitamin B_{12} produced better-quality embryos.[21]

Similarly, researchers in Italy have found high levels of CoQ_{10}, a molecule found in just about every cell in the body and critical to preserving egg quality and fertility, in ovarian follicles containing high-quality eggs and in eggs that became high-quality embryos.[22] CoQ_{10} is believed to improve egg quality by helping eggs to produce more energy, which is critically important to an egg's ability to successfully complete the process of meiosis. As women age, the mitochondria in their eggs becomes less efficient at producing the energy needed to mature and fertilize, perhaps the single most determinative factor in egg and embryo quality.[23] CoQ_{10}, importantly, improves mitochondrial function and protects mitochondria from damage,[24] enabling an egg to have a far greater chance of growing and dividing successfully.

Simply taking a prenatal vitamin including these important B vitamins and CoQ_{10} during the months before conception can substantially increase the odds of conception and decrease the odds of miscarriage. Women like Sharon and Stacy are great believers. After five years of unsuccessful fertility treatments following her first baby, Sharon turned to multivitamins and acupuncture and conceived naturally, giving birth to a beautiful, healthy boy. Stacy likewise conceived after giving up on IVF following multiple failed attempts, turning instead toward a more natural approach—multivitamins, acupuncture, and eliminating toxins like BPA. She now has a gorgeous, healthy girl.

Bisphenol A, or BPA, found in a great many plastics, such as water bottles and food containers as well as paper receipts, is a fertility disaster. Numerous studies illuminate the devastating effects of BPA on fertility,[25] not to mention the hundreds of studies over the last fifteen years that point to the toxic effects of BPA on diabetes, heart disease, liver failure, and obesity. Women with high levels of BPA have lower estrogen levels (estrogen is needed to stimulate ovarian follicles to grow), fewer eggs, a lower fertilization rate for those eggs, and fewer fertilized embryos implanting in the uterus—all factors that create enormous challenges to a woman trying to conceive.[26] A group of researchers at the Harvard T. H. Chan School of Public Health found that the impact of BPA on getting pregnant was so significant that the quartile of women with the highest BPA exposure had only *half* as much chance of an embryo implanting as the quartile with the lowest BPA exposure.[27] Crucially, BPA also impedes normal cell division during meiosis, leading to severe chromosomal abnormalities, and has been shown to interfere with stimulation protocols and egg development in women undergoing IVF.[28]

Not surprisingly, given the impact of BPA on egg quality, studies in the United States[29] and Japan[30] also indicate that BPA raises the risk of miscarriage. In one study, where pregnant women with fertility challenges (either trouble getting pregnant, a history of miscarriage, or both) were separated into four groups based on the level of BPA in their blood serum, it was found that the women with the highest levels of BPA had an 80 percent greater likelihood of miscarriage than those with the lowest levels. Even tiny amounts of BPA distort hormonal systems and damage eggs, decreasing the chances of conception and increasing rates of miscarriage.

Frighteningly, the impact of BPA may be multigenerational. Because fetal exposure may damage all the immature egg cells in a developing female, "the implications for human fertility are profound."[31] Not only is a daughter of a woman exposed to BPA at risk, but if the daughter's eggs are all affected, her future children may be at risk too. Unfortunately, because the potential disturbances occur in utero, any impact on the offspring will not become evident until the children reach maturity, making a clear connection between cause and effect a daunting task.

But importantly, the effects of BPA on the body are temporary. Eliminating or minimizing exposure to BPA will swiftly lower the amount of BPA in the system. Given the impact of BPA during the all-important time of meiosis, it can be extremely beneficial to limit exposure during the months before trying to conceive. Simple things like throwing out plastic containers (yes, including bottled water!), avoiding hot food packaged in plastic, washing hands after handling receipts, and choosing shampoos and cosmetics that are BPA free, particularly in the weeks and months before ovulation, can increase the odds of a healthy baby.

In her book, *It Starts with the Egg*, Rebecca Fett describes her journey from her diagnosis of diminished ovarian reserve to the mother of a healthy baby. Not yet thirty years old when she was diagnosed and told she faced very low odds of producing healthy eggs, Rebecca followed a comprehensive, scientific "self-help" approach, taking daily supplements, eliminating plastics and other toxins, and altering her diet. In only a few months, she increased the number of eggs developing in her ovaries from just a handful to over twenty, nineteen of which eventually fertilized and grew to the blastocyst stage—rendering a record for her prestigious fertility clinic. She and her husband opted to transfer only one blastocyst, resulting in the birth of her beautiful, healthy son.

Similarly, my friend Susan, who had experienced multiple IVF failures with very low egg counts when attempting to conceive her second child in her late thirties, pursued a program of vitamins and eliminating toxins, together with acupuncture and traditional Chinese medicine, improving her egg quality so radically that she conceived naturally.

Low Dosage or "Mini" and Natural-Cycle IVF

"Far too little proper research is being done to improve IVF. We are very complacent," said IVF pioneer Lord Winston in 2008, noting the disappointing lack of improvement in IVF success rates over several decades. Observing that even the lackluster success rate of around 30 percent was possible only because doctors were "picking the right patients to treat," Lord Winston concluded: "I can see in five to ten years time at most, new therapies to produce eggs which are much more likely to be viable and the embryos quality depends on the quality of the egg."[32]

Nearly nine years later, many experts agree with Lord Winston, and there is mounting evidence that conventional IVF stimulation may not be the best way forward—at least not in all cases. "We have created an enormously wasteful system," Dr. Bart Fauser, chair of the department of reproductive medicine and gynecology at University Medical Center Utrecht, declared at an international conference of expert scientists and doctors.[33] "Not all eggs are created equal," the widely cited Dutch specialist continued, explaining that eggs come from very different follicles and very different stages of development. In response to the idea that the more eggs you start out with, the more good ones you will get: "It is not that simple," he concluded. "Embryo quality is very complex."

An IVF cycle has many variables contributing to its eventual success or failure. While the generation of eggs is clearly key, it is not the only ingredient needed for a winning recipe. The egg must develop into a healthy embryo and then implant. The ovarian stimulation protocols used in IVF do not only have implications for the quality of the eggs, but also for the endometrium, or endometrial lining, which lines the uterus, and which typically thickens throughout the menstrual cycle in preparation for receiving a fertilized egg. In addition to the higher rates of chromosomal abnormalities seen in the embryos of stimulated cycles, as many as half of all embryos transferred do not implant, suggesting that it is not only the quality of the embryo that is important to conception but also a uterine lining ready to provide a hospitable environment.

I experienced the problems of a thinning endometrium firsthand, as my uterine lining dwindled in successive IVF cycles, to the point that it reached a mere four to five millimeters in my last few attempts in London, far short of the minimum eight to ten millimeters hoped for by my doctors. When they added Viagra to my drug cocktail, my lining increased slightly to six millimeters, still short of the goal. But I was simply told that, among my many challenges, I had a thin lining. I had no idea that my repeat high-dosage IVF cycles might be causing or contributing to the thin lining.

Due to the falloff in numbers at every stage of the process, it takes nearly twenty oocytes (immature egg cells) to generate one live birth using conventional IVF. Yet interestingly, two studies found limits to the optimal number of eggs retrieved. The first showed that retrievals of more than ten eggs produced lower-quality eggs and lower fertility rates than retrievals of ten or fewer eggs. The latter study showed a similar fall in pregnancy rates when more than thirteen eggs were retrieved in a given cycle.[34]

"The US is much more aggressive than Europe in obtaining eggs," Dr. Jacques Cohen declared.[35] Educated in Holland, Dr. Cohen, a renowned embryologist who began his career at Bourn Hall Clinic, the world's first IVF clinic, is director of the ART Institute of Washington as well as director and cofounder of Reprogenetics. Sometimes this aggressive approach is better, he explained, but not always. Acknowledging the potential impact on embryo quality, aneuploidy, and the endometrium, experts in much of the world are moving toward using the lowest effective dosages in treating their patients. For example, highlighting the lack of evidence that higher dosages of stimulation help people have children, Dr. Zion Ben-Rafael, one of Israel's leading fertility experts and founder and chairman of the World Congress on Controversies in Obstetrics, Gynecology & Infertility, emphasized that the use of any dosage higher than 300 to 350 IUs of gonadotropins should be questioned, urging his colleagues to in fact lower the doses if a patient is responding well. Those like Dr. Oxana, Dr. Ben-Rafael, Dr. Fauser, and a host of others, believe we can get better results in IVF with fewer drugs, less intervention, and yes, fewer eggs.

Low dosage or "mini" IVF aims to do exactly that. Focusing, as the New Hope Fertility Center in New York City aptly states, on "quality over quantity," low-dosage IVF seeks to stimulate a far smaller number of eggs with ideally less disruption to the system. As Dr. Oxana first told me in Moscow, it takes only one good egg to make a baby, and that egg is more likely to be obtained with fewer external threats to its natural development. Although mini IVF protocols vary, ranging from clinics that use only Clomid or letrozole for stimulation to those that use Clomid in combination with several days of low-dose (150 IU) gonadotropin injections to those, like mine, that included over a week of low-dose injections, the goal is generally to produce in the range of three to five eggs, a higher proportion of which is expected to be normal.

Mini IVF offers certain advantages for patients, not the least of which is financial. Lower dosages of hormones over fewer days results in fewer side effects, quicker cycles, and lower costs, without reducing pregnancy rates per embryo transfer. The promise of an easier cycle is no small thing: when I tried the lower dose IVF, I was certain that it wasn't working because I didn't feel a thing. No tension headaches. No bloating. No irritability (my polite way of saying I was a crazy person about to snap at any moment). And its success rates are impressive. Dutch researchers found higher ongoing pregnancy rates per embryo transfer with mild stimulation.[36] A Spanish study found significant increases in rates of fertilization and chromosomally normal blastocysts in reduced-dose IVF cycles.[37] A Russian team similarly found higher numbers of chromosomal abnormalities among eggs subject to conventional controlled ovarian stimulation than those without.[38]

In use in other countries for more than a decade, it is finally starting to catch on in the United States, albeit at very few clinics, due to the distinct benefits it offers: a higher proportion of chromosomally normal embryos than that of conventional IVF, fewer mosaics, lower risk of ovarian hyperstimulation, reduced impact on the uterine lining (important for implantation), and lower risk of multiples.[39] In perhaps the first randomized controlled study in the United States, Dr. Zhang and his team at New Hope Fertility Center assigned 564 women to either a mini IVF group, which underwent single embryo transfers, or a conventional IVF group, which experienced double embryo transfers. The cumulative live birth rate was 49 percent for the mini IVF group compared to 63 percent for the conventional group, but the mini IVF group had no cases of ovarian hyperstimulation compared with sixteen cases, or 5.7 percent, of moderate to severe hyperstimulation in the conventional group. Additionally, the mini IVF group experienced a multiple pregnancy rate of only 6.4 percent, as compared to 32 percent for the conventional group, at a far lower cost per cycle.[40] While costs vary between clinics, mini IVF in the United States typically costs approximately $5,000 to $7,500 per cycle, which can be *two to four times less* than the cost of conventional IVF. So while the success rate per cycle (although not per embryo) may be lower, some women, particularly those with polycystic ovaries who are at higher risk of ovarian hyperstimulation, or those with low ovarian reserve, may prefer the less expensive, less invasive protocol that can be repeated in back-to-back cycles.

Going one step—or perhaps a leap—further than mini IVF is the practice of natural cycle IVF. Natural cycle IVF, pioneered in Japan more than twenty years ago, involves removing an egg in an unstim-ulated cycle. No Clomid, no hormone shots. In the vast majority of these cycles, one egg is obtained through the egg retrieval—a "one shot" situation I imagine would be stressful for a good deal of women and couples. But I was amazed to discover how well those solo embryos could do. The live birth rate per embryo for women under thirty-five was 26.6 percent using natural IVF, as compared to 20.6 percent using mini IVF and 4.3 percent using conventional (high-dose) stimulation protocols. That's nearly four times higher than conventional IVF! The overall success rates, not surprisingly, were lower among older women, but the correlations remained the same; for women aged thirty-eight to forty, for example, the natural stimulation group had live birth rates of 13.6 percent per embryo compared to 10.6 percent and 3.1 percent for the mini and conventional IVF groups, respectively.[41]

These statistics do not address the fact that it may take many cycles to achieve success with natural IVF, and that in stimulated IVF there is a bigger pool of embryos from which to choose. But the implication seems clear: an egg obtained without the typical high-dose gonadotro-pins is more likely to be viable than one obtained through conventional ovarian stimulation, and has a greater chance of becoming a live baby.

Critics of both low-dose and natural IVF argue that these methods are not for everyone, contending that many women will end up with no embryos to transfer and insisting that higher numbers of eggs are needed to find the viable ones.

But the point is: there are options. And it is important to ask about them and to assess what makes the most sense in each individual case. Identify specific problems. Understand that there are different paths.

For certain categories of women, such as those with polycystic ova-ries, like me, who have a tendency to produce high numbers of eggs and are at risk of ovarian hyperstimulation syndrome, or who—also like me—experience irregular or absent ovulation, or those with endo-metriosis or a low ovarian reserve, low-dose IVF seems to make a lot of sense. It is certainly worth discussing with a specialist. Others may require higher levels of stimulation. If there is one thing I have learned through my own experience, as well as my encounters with numerous others, it is that no one size fits all in confronting infertility.

Improving Egg Quality through Hormones: The Pregmama Story

"What if we could use hormones to actually make eggs healthier inside the woman? Improve egg quality and possibly eliminate the need for IVF in some cases?" Dr. Lori Bernstein's enthusiasm came through on the phone, and I was excited too. A medical way to cure aging eggs?

Dr. Bernstein's interest is both personal and professional. A doctor of biology educated at Johns Hopkins University and Harvard College, Dr. Bernstein and her husband easily conceived six times but miscarried each time. Her seventh pregnancy happily was a charm, and she gave birth to their healthy, beloved baby daughter. But when they tried to conceive a sibling for their daughter, she was back on the treadmill of losses. After nine pregnancies, Dr. Bernstein and her husband had one daughter, lots of heartache, and also lots of data. They had tested the remains from many of her miscarriages, and each one had chromosomal abnormalities. Driven by an intellectual desire to understand the root causes of egg aneuploidy as well as an emotional desire to help others have babies, she decided to switch her professional focus from cancer research to reproductive endocrinology and egg biology.

"We have to overcome the dogma," Dr. Bernstein told me when we first spoke. She is now the founder and chief scientific officer of Pregmama, LLC as well as an adjunct professor at the University of Maryland School of Medicine and at Texas A&M University College of Veterinary Medicine & Biomedical Sciences. "The 'eggs can't be cured' dogma . . . the 'inherent aging problem with eggs' dogma," she explains.

It is one thing to acknowledge that environmental influences affect egg quality, and that conventional ovarian stimulation protocols designed to help women have healthy babies may, ironically, in some cases, be harming the tiny eggs they are designed to help. It is another step to accept that removing these influences, even after years of exposure, may foster an environment that enables the maturation of healthy eggs. But it is a greater leap still to establish that there may be a medical protocol that an infertile woman can administer at home that can "cure" her eggs, enabling her to conceive. This is the leap that Dr. Bernstein and her team are making.

It is well-known that as women age, their supply of eggs diminishes. When they have fewer eggs, their inhibin level goes down. Inhibin is a protein that suppresses FSH, so when a woman's inhibin level drops, her FSH level goes up. Although most clinicians firmly believe that FSH levels have no bearing on whether embryos have a normal complement of chromosomes, Dr. Bernstein begs to differ, noting that this conclusion is not justified by the data. Referring to studies that demonstrate that high levels of FSH strongly correlate to high numbers of embryos with trisomy, she argues that this clear correlation supports the hypothesis that high FSH is a cause of aneuploidy, particularly among older women.

Dr. Bernstein founded Pregmama to develop protocols to reduce FSH levels among women and thereby help cure their infertility. Together with her colleagues, Dr. Bernstein performed studies on midlife mice with elevated FSH, high rates of egg aneuploidy, and diminished fertility.[42] When they lowered the FSH levels in the mice through treatment, the quality of their eggs increased, chromosome abnormalities decreased, and fertility significantly improved. Conversely, increasing FSH levels in the mice led to dramatically increased rates of chromosome abnormalities and reduced fertility.

Her goals are admittedly ambitious: "To bring babies into the world. To prevent egg aneuploidy and embryo death in AMA [advanced maternal age] women.[43] [To reduce] the incidence of infertility, miscarriage and/or trisomic stillborns and live-borns."[44] Dr. Bernstein's research is deeply rooted in the (scientifically supported) belief that hormone levels have an impact on egg quality. While recent research has looked at the impact of external hormones, such as the IVF injections, on egg and embryo quality, it is a woman's internal environment, her natural hormone levels, that intrigues her. Acknowledging that the "notion that hormone levels in women may cause oocyte aneuploidy has been largely discarded by obstetricians and gynecologists," Dr. Bernstein has a different perspective. Citing data that supports her hypothesis that it is hormonal aging that plays an important role in causing errors in meiosis, and therefore in egg and embryo quality, she believes it is possible to reduce the incidence of chromosome abnormalities in older women or those with fertility challenges by restoring the hormone balance to that of a young, fertile woman.

Dr. Bernstein's first therapy, now in clinical trials, is called Veriploid, and she and her team are already at work on a second method called Eggtivin. "Veriploid is designed to roll back the clock to enable healthy egg maturation, meaning an egg with the correct number of chromosomes," said Dr. Bernstein. Although still in the trial stage, Pregmama's Veriploid therapy has already achieved its first pregnancy and live birth. A healthy baby boy was born in January 2016 to a forty-five-year-old woman who had experienced five years of infertility before agreeing to join the trial.

The treatment comprises drugs that have been used safely for many years in other medical contexts. The key difference here is the dosage, and the length of time a woman takes them. The idea of the treatment is to bring the FSH closer to its ideal levels, in order to create a cellular environment that fosters the growth and maturation of healthy, chromosomally normal eggs that may be capable of becoming fertilized naturally. Imagine that. Having a kit at home to self-administer hormones, which are carefully monitored and adjusted, and even getting pregnant the old-fashioned way.

Too good to be true? Dr. Bernstein doesn't think so.

Tomorrow belongs only to the people who prepare for it today.

Malcolm X

14

Minding the Gaps

Reflections on the Future of Fertility

S*eeing* my beautiful, healthy children playing joyfully with their new (naturally conceived) baby cousin, I wonder if my daughter, in particular, will confront the challenges I faced in trying to have her own children. Did she inherit my hormone imbalances? My challenging immune system? My arcuate uterus? If so, what will treatment look like two to three decades from now? Will she be able to afford it? Will she have the critical information she will need to make informed decisions? Will the entire landscape have changed in ways I can't even imagine?

My children, like the children of so many amazing people whom I have met in the process of writing this book, would not be here today without the incredible advances made by scientists and doctors over the past half century. Paula and Derrick's twins; Pietro and Peter's daughter;

Robert and Jeffrey's twins; my own Alexandra and William. They would all be just figments of our imaginations rather than the living, breathing human beings we so cherish.

Since the birth of Louise Brown, pioneering physicians have refined IVF techniques and protocols; embryologists have invented new culture mediums and greatly enhanced our understanding of embryo development and the ability of embryos to survive in the lab; geneticists have developed ever-more-accurate techniques to assess the chromosomal makeup of eggs and embryos; and the further evolution and acceptance of IVF have enabled parents in need of assistance to enlist the aid of egg donors, sperm donors, and surrogates in their quest to have a child. Indeed, for would-be parents who know how to ask the right questions and access the necessary information, there are now a myriad of treatment options available—if they can pay for those treatments, or are fortunate to live in one of the rare states with adequate insurance coverage available (or better yet, in a country with national insurance).

Yet regrettably, despite many laudable advances, significant gaps persist in the United States in the provision of nearly every aspect of fertility treatment, limiting our ability to treat those in need in the most effective, efficient, and fair manner. There is a gap between the costs of treatment and the amount most people can afford to pay; a gap between the fruits of scientific research and the understanding and treatment options offered by many, if not most, practitioners to their patients; and a gap between the life-giving possibilities that are quickly evolving with the advent of new technologies and the policies and laws in place that govern not only the provision of fertility services but also the recognition of parenthood itself. In order to take advantage of the many remarkable advances in treating infertility and increase availability to all who desire and would benefit from the advances, we need to close these gaps.

The Financial Gap

The stark reality is that in America, in 2016, overcoming infertility is only for the rich, and the lucky few who live in Connecticut, Illinois, Maryland, Massachusetts, New Jersey, or one of the other few states that require insurers to cover, at least to some extent, IVF. In a country in which only one-third of the population has $1,000 or more available to them in an emergency, the high costs of IUI, IVF, and other fertility advances clearly leave many who require them in need. Those who can afford expert advice, IVF at the best clinics, expensive egg donors if need be, the fees charged by legitimate agencies, compensation for surrogates if necessary, and legal fees, are much more likely to have the baby they dream of than those who cannot.

But it doesn't need to be this way. Those seeking fertility assistance in Canada, Australia, Sweden, Spain, France, Denmark, the Netherlands, even Saudi Arabia, don't face this first, often prohibitive, obstacle. In these nations, and a host of others, infertility is considered a medical problem like diabetes or cancer, and treatments that aim to address it are covered by the national health system as with any other disease. Moreover, their free or highly subsidized care is often accompanied by live birth rates that rival those of some of the expensive clinics in the United States. Many insurance carriers in the United States, in contrast, not required by federal law to treat it as they treat other medical conditions, tend to regard infertility as a social issue—an elective procedure—rather than a medical one. As is the case with elective plastic surgery, for example, insurance companies often deny coverage altogether, or perhaps allow patients to purchase supplemental coverage as an "add-on." Yet few women "elect" being infertile.

Given the current political climate, in which the Affordable Care Act and Medicare seem perilously at risk, it is difficult to imagine the type of broad sweeping support of fertility treatment in the United States that is a given in other developed countries, but as with the provision of health care generally, I believe there is a moral imperative to treat aspiring parents more evenly throughout society. Do we want to live in a country where affluent, predominantly white people confronting infertility are able to afford the medical teams and treatments they need to help them have a baby, while their less financially secure neighbors cannot? A country where those fortunate to live in a state like Illinois, which covers IVF, may sit side by side in a fertility clinic waiting room with counterparts from Wisconsin, only 5 percent of whom have insurance that covers IVF? Imagine the frustration of women who live in a state like New York, which requires that insurers cover diagnostic tests such as hysterosalpingograms, endometrial biopsies, blood tests, and ultrasounds—all given in order to detect *medical* problems—but does not mandate that those insurers provide coverage for procedures such as IVF to remedy the fertility problems that the tests may reveal.[1]

Insurance is shaping treatments in ways that are neither best for the patient nor financially sound—often leading women, for example, to transfer higher numbers of embryos in hopes of avoiding another cycle, mandating treatment at certain clinics and prohibiting it at others, and forgoing testing that could help ensure against abnormalities. Even in "good states," like Massachusetts, insurance coverage can be maddeningly inconsistent. Nina, the physician in Boston, and her husband, Ken, felt fortunate to live in Massachusetts, where their insurance covered IVF treatments. Indeed, Nina recalls laughing when they discovered that their insurance would pay for six cycles, which seemed to them like a very high number.

"We thought there was no way we would ever be in the position of trying IVF six times," she told me. "I thought I would give up way before then. But you wake up one day, and you are there."

Embarking on their adventure full of hope, Nina did not anticipate the cycle of pregnancy and miscarriage that was to follow. Almost paralleling my history, she experienced five miscarriages, all naturally conceived, four of which resulted from chromosomal abnormalities. Complicating her situation, Ken had a mitochondrial disorder, and the doctors had no idea whether this was playing a role. After three failed IVF cycles, neither Nina, Ken, nor their doctors felt it wise to continue IVF without genetic testing that would identify any normal embryos. The physical and emotional toll was just too high. Their insurance company, however, wouldn't pay for the testing. It would cover three more cycles of IVF, at approximately $15,000 a pop, but would not cover $3,000 for the genetic testing that might take them off their dreadful treadmill. In order to get the testing they and their doctors believed was necessary, they paid out of pocket. Coincidentally, Nina's sister, at virtually the same time, was also trying to conceive in Massachusetts. She learned that she and her husband were carriers of Canavan disease, a recessive degenerative disorder that causes damage to nerve cells in the brain, and that any child they might have had a one in four chance of having Canavan as well. Their Massachusetts insurance covered up to six cycles of IVF with PGD. Nina has yet to have a child, while her sister, with the help of IVF with PGD, gave birth to a healthy girl.

Given this uneven and complicated landscape, what is a woman or couple confronting infertility or recurrent miscarriage to do? Or a gay couple or single woman who desires to have a child? As things stand now, in the absence of deep resources, the best people can do is to try to game the system:

Get as many tests covered by insurance as possible. Even in states without mandated fertility coverage, basic diagnostic procedures, such as blood tests and ultrasounds, which can shed a great deal of light on fertility problems, will often be covered.

Shop around for fertility drugs. When living in London, I ordered my IVF medicines (after a cycle that was completely funded by the National Health Service) from a group called the International Pharmacy Organisation, which delivered them directly to me at prices far lower than those offered by my New York clinic. Some Americans save money by ordering their medications online either domestically or looking to countries such as Canada, Israel, or the United Kingdom.[2]

Look for a job with a company that covers infertility treatment. Seriously, for some, this is the answer. Go work for Spotify, Bank of America, Discovery Communications, Time Warner, Chanel, Intel, Apple, Facebook, Perkins Coie, Zappos, and a host of other companies that provide excellent fertility care. Job switching for fertility benefits has become common enough to spark web forums, such as "Jobs With Infertility Coverage";[3] coverage in mainstream media like *Fortune*;[4] and a shout-out in FertilityIQ,[5] a company whose raison d'être is to help patients navigate the infertility treatment maze. Although just over a quarter of employers in America provide infertility coverage, the number is growing, led in large part by technology companies that are pouring more money into fertility benefits than any other industry in an effort to attract and retain talent and create a work environment where working parents and aspiring parents can thrive. Recognizing that "the impact [fertility] benefit[s] can have on an employee's life is immeasurable," Southwest Airlines now offers partial coverage to its team members, more than one hundred of whom use the benefit annually.[6]

Talk to doctors about protocols that maximize the return on dollars spent. Patients may wish to consider financial considerations in shaping their treatment plan. Mini IVF, for example, which requires the purchase of far fewer drugs as well as lower cycle costs, may be an appropriate course to pursue for many women. Given the low success rates of IUI, raise the question of skipping the usual three cycles of IUI before moving on to IVF, potentially saving time and money in the process. In the same vein, although PGS may seem to add to the costs of IVF, it could potentially eliminate the need for follow-on cycles.

Consider traveling to lower-cost places. Jenny went to Spain; Sandra went to Mexico; I went to Russia. Articles abound of couples traveling to Israel, India, Thailand, and, more recently, Argentina and Barbados. Fertility tourism, or reprotravel, may offer a viable solution for those with the time, ability, and appetite for travel. Treatment in some of these countries is offered at costs less than the cost of the drugs in the United States, while maintaining high success rates. A cycle of IVF costs on average $6,000 in Spain, $7,800 in Mexico, $3,300 in India, and $3,000 in Russia, as opposed to $12,000 to $25,000 in the United States.[7]

There is much work to be done to make quality infertility care affordable to a far greater percentage of the population, but in the meantime, there are steps individuals can take to improve their access to the best care available. It is imperative that fertility patients get informed about their own challenges and the paths available to them. Be aware that a purchaser of infertility care is a consumer, not just a patient, and must approach the acquisition of fertility treatment to some degree as one would any other significant purchase. One IVF cycle in the United States costs as much as a car. Doesn't it deserve as much research effort?

The Information Gap

Paula spent hours, days, late nights, bent over her computer researching her own fertility problems, intent on understanding them and having a say in her care. Likewise, Jessica, with the help of her physician husband, invested so much time educating herself on all aspects of her fertility care that it became her "secret second job." Marcy, Susan, and I, all lawyers, attacked our problems as we would a complex legal problem, tracking down every available piece of information and analyzing it from all angles.

Reflecting on my numerous conversations with these amazingly persistent women, I realize that there is a common thread beyond, for some of us, a JD. We all sought to educate ourselves about our challenges, outside the sphere of what our doctors told us. Of course, we all sought and received medical advice from our doctors, and much of it was helpful, but, despite being in different cities with different doctors and different problems, we each came to the same conclusion: that the information we had been given was insufficient; that the protocols were not necessarily tailored to our individual situations; that we were rarely presented with options. Instinctively, we all knew that we weren't being given the full story—that there must be something more.

The instinct, especially in the age of instant information, to google medical problems is certainly not limited to sussing out infertility. When I painfully damaged my knee, tearing my ACL and meniscus, my orthopedist told me that I needed to have surgery and suggested a cadaver graft. I promptly went to the Internet, not because I didn't believe what he was saying but because I wanted to learn about the surgery and understand what it entailed. I read the views of others who had been through it, digesting the pros and cons of using a cadaver versus my own patellar tendon. Nothing I read contradicted what my orthopedic specialist told me, and I did not question his judgment; I simply wanted to supplement his advice and prepare myself for the long recovery.

It does not feel the same, however, with the quest for knowledge about fertility treatments. Although I, like virtually everyone with whom I spoke, started out regarding my fertility problems like any other medical issue, relying on the advice of my doctor, over time I became increasingly dubious. It is virtually impossible to pinpoint precisely when that begins to happen, but one day you wake up and realize that you don't exactly trust what you are being told. Something just doesn't feel right. Some, like Jessica and Paula, felt that their doctors, focused on numbers and success rates and profitability, pushed them toward certain protocols. Rose and Anna viewed their own clinics as too standardized, failing to differentiate the protocols to account for their individual situations. Marcy found her first clinic to be so protective of its own success rate that they didn't want to treat a difficult case.

Underlying their differing resentments was the shared sense that they simply didn't receive enough accurate information about the available treatment options, the probability of failure, or the costs. And, perhaps because emotions run high when discussing experiences at fertility clinics, no patient I spoke to attributed this lack of disclosure to a benign cause. All seemed to feel there was a willful withholding of information. But is it that simple?

In an almost complicit relationship between doctor and patient, doctors are perceived to be all-knowing. The patient goes to a doctor, particularly a specialist, with the expectation that a problem will be solved. Fertility experts try their best to provide solutions and often rely on what has worked before. Patients tend to follow their advice unquestioningly, even when they are uneasy. I know I did. I deferred to the experts. Yet our understanding of egg and embryo development, the role of hormones, endometrial lining, genetic testing, culture mediums, oxygen levels in incubators and other factors is constantly evolving, contributing to a widening gap between the knowledge gained through scientific research and medical practice. Fertility specialists running extremely busy clinics (and businesses), in a vacuum of federal regulation, are not necessarily keeping up with the advances or incorporating them in their practice. Add to that a further communication gap between the knowledge of doctors and what they impart to their patients. Whether the knowledge gap is intentional or accidental, most patients feel that salient information is not filtering down the chain.

On the more cynical end of the spectrum, experts within the field have noted that it's not in the interest of fertility doctors to make their treatments more effective, that there is "almost a willingness to remain ignorant" as it is "easier and more lucrative to keep doing the same old thing"; that having people "fail means that they come back again."[8] Slightly less pessimistic, scientists I spoke with at the conferences I attended attributed the small number of fertility doctors present, particularly those from the United States, as stemming either from arrogance or complacency. "They already have the biggest market, the world flocking to them, regardless of their success rates, so they don't feel the need to change their methods," one European embryologist wryly commented, noting that clinicians often give patients wrong, or outdated advice. When I asked why, he responded that the current information is "not what's in their grasp." Another explanation is that they are simply too busy treating patients to take time off for conferences, a rationale that seems to extend to the doctor-patient relationship as well. Among the many patients I spoke with who felt grossly underinformed by their doctors, the perception was that the doctors were either too busy, or too paternalistic, to have the detailed exchange of information they desired.

Whatever the reasons, there seems to be an unacceptable culture of ignorance permeating the communication chain. Patients need accurate and current information in order to make the right decisions about their fertility options. But if they are not getting the whole story from their doctors, where are they going to get it?

More and more, they are getting it from one other, and for the hearty few, from publications aimed at those in the medical field. For many years, fertility patients have built networks aimed at offering emotional support and the sharing of valued practical information. Communities like those formed around Resolve: The National Infertility Association, Fertility Authority, FertileThoughts, Fertility.org, and Fertility Friends provide not only emotional support from those in the same shoes but also often include detailed descriptions of treatments (what hurts, what doesn't), protocols (what works, what doesn't), clinics and doctors (who's good, who's not), and even specific travel information for those considering reproductive tourism abroad.

Recently, after tackling the unexpectedly difficult task of finding the best fertility doctor and clinic for themselves—navigating a maze "filled with hearsay, half-truths, and marketing spin" as well as frustrating and potentially harmful medical errors—Jake and Deborah Anderson-Bialis founded FertilityIQ, a website dedicated to compiling crowd-sourced data to help fertility patients educate themselves and make decisions on their care.[9] Focused initially on compiling evaluations by patients of doctors and clinics to help others select the right doctor for them, FertilityIQ now also offers extensive data on expenses; insurance coverage; companies with good insurance plans; IVF success rates by occupation, educational level, wealth, and geography; as well as expert commentary on the medical aspects of fertility treatment—essentially a Bloomberg for fertility. Not surprisingly, in examining how IVF patients feel about the quality of information they receive in the treatment process, the FertilityIQ team discovered that nearly half of all patients surveyed regard IVF as the most important moment in their lives, yet *nearly three-quarters feel that the information they receive is insufficient* and half worry that it is biased.[10]

For those willing to plunge into more detailed scientific information, *Fertility and Sterility,* an international journal for various specialists treating and investigating infertility and reproductive disorders, proved to be an invaluable source of information on my specific problems. Though not exactly beach reading, I found most articles to be quite clear and very helpful.

An aspiring parent is well served to talk to people, peruse websites, question doctors, read scientific journals, look at international sources. It doesn't matter how one gets one's information, but it is essential to get the information needed to make an informed decision. Information is power, and key to success.

The Policy Gap

What makes a parent a parent? Who is entitled to be called a parent? The person who provides the genetic material (even in the case of a donor who has agreed to donate and give up parental rights)? The woman who carries the baby (even in the case of gestational surrogacy where she has no genetic connection to the baby)? The individuals who commissioned the birth (even if one or both intended parents is not a genetic parent)?

Who is entitled to determine the fate of an embryo once created? One of the parents? Both the parents? What if they disagree? In the case of donation, is the "parent" the donor or the intended parent?

Is it morally acceptable to select an embryo for certain traits, like gender? To create a baby who is a perfect genetic match to save the life of another? Once possible, to manipulate an embryo for certain traits through gene editing?

Scientific advancement has given rise to a host of extremely difficult ethical questions that our society has yet to deal with in any way that closely approximates a consistent and holistic manner. The government, for the most part, is of little help in addressing these challenges, and the regulations that do exist are haphazard at best.

I don't believe that the federal legislators who failed to regulate IVF in the 1970s; or the current state legislators in states like New York and Michigan that prohibit or criminalize surrogacy, or in states like Georgia, Maine, or Hawaii that fail to regulate it at all; or the legislators in Illinois who permit embryo donation subject to contract while judges in Massachusetts have found such contracts to be unenforceable, intended to create a Rubik's Cube in which those who can solve the puzzle (and afford it) can purchase the desired fertility services in a favorable jurisdiction, while those who cannot (and lack the financial resources) remain childless. Yet unfortunately, that is where we find ourselves today.

Would-be parents formerly incapable of having children can now achieve their dreams through a myriad of ways previously reserved for the province of science fiction: single women or lesbian couples can use a sperm donor; single men or gay couples can turn to an egg donor and surrogate; straight couples facing infertility can try IUI, IVF, IVF with PGS or PGD, ICSI, and, if necessary, donation or surrogacy. But to legally claim parenthood of these miracle babies, the intended parents must reside, or conceive, or give birth, as the case may be, in the right place. If Catherine, our practically perfect surrogate, had given birth to Alexandra and William in New York rather than England, she would have been deemed their mother and I would have had to adopt my own children, presuming I was lucky enough for her not to challenge my motherhood.

Even more complicated are the rules surrounding the use of embryos, particularly with respect to the field of embryo donation, also, somewhat controversially, known as embryo adoption. Regulations relating to frozen embryo usage and embryo donation are so inconsistent that they make the patchwork quilt of rules regarding egg and sperm donation and surrogacy look downright organized. Since there is no central repository of information about frozen embryos, it is difficult to know with certainty, but experts estimate that there are likely about a million embryos in storage today.[11]

Usually frozen by couples or singles intending to save them for future cycles, whether as backup for a failed cycle or for a theoretical sibling, most people are not focused on the ultimate disposition of their unused embryos at the time of their creation. Options such as disposing of them, donating them for research, or giving them to another family hoping to have a child, raise questions for many about the moral and legal status of the embryo. Philosophical and personal views can become oddly intertwined, and conflicting. Harkening uncomfortably close to the abortion debate, for example, some question when life begins, and whether destroying an embryo is destroying a life. While most couples avoid addressing such issues at the outset, even those who initially come to a decision often change their minds after the embryos have been created, as they may begin to think of them as their own frozen children. Couples who initially planned to donate to another family may feel differently when confronted with the reality of giving their hard-earned embryo away, finding the idea of another genetic child out in the world, a biological sibling to their own son or daughter, a bit too uncomfortable. With substantial numbers of people unable to decide or agree, the national stock of embryos builds. Even those who think they are clear are often reluctant to act. Richard and I have always agreed that we would donate our embryos to research, and we still plan to do so. But we haven't gotten around to doing it yet. Most of the patients I interviewed had a clear plan, but no one I spoke with has actually disposed or transferred their embryos.

While there is rarely conflict when the embryos are used in a future cycle as envisioned, there is plenty of room for disagreement when it comes to what to do with the embryos that are not used as planned in a subsequent cycle for the same intended parent(s). Couples who separate after the embryos are frozen, for example, face questions about their embryos' fate. In 2015, Nick Loeb, formerly engaged to Sofia Vergara, publicly called out the "important questions about life, religion, and parenthood" raised by embryonic custody disputes in an op-ed arguing that a man "who is willing to take on all parental responsibilities [should] be . . . entitled to bring his embryos to term even if the woman objects."[12] Acknowledging that the couple signed a form stating that any embryos could be brought to life only with both parties' consent, Loeb contends that the form did not comply with California law, which requires that the couple specify what would happen in the event of separation, and should therefore be voided. Vergara, now married to another man and not interested in having a child with her ex-fiancé, wants the embryos to remain frozen. Their case, like others, is now in the hands of the state court system, where judges have been generally reluctant to compel a person to become a parent against her or his will; the few exceptions to date have arisen in cases in which the potential mothers had undergone chemotherapy rendering their frozen embryos the only means by which each could become a biological parent, tipping the balancing of interests in favor of the woman's desire to have a child over the man's desire not to procreate.[13]

Perhaps the only issue dicier than deciding custody of existing frozen embryos is the question of regulating the creation of embryos expressly for donation, whether for research or for "adoption." Scientific research on embryos has long been a hotbed of controversy, with the United States, not surprisingly, as an outlier on the more restrictive end of the spectrum. While only a handful of European countries, including Belgium, Sweden, and the United Kingdom, permit the creation of embryos for research, most European nations allow research on donated embryos left over from IVF cycles. Since 1995, federal regulation in the United States has banned funding of any research that involves destruction of an embryo, whether existing or created for research purposes. But private funding and certain state laws have sought to fill in the gap, with eight states enacting policies that encourage embryonic research, in contrast with an almost equal number that prohibit or severely restrict it.[14]

Ironically, at the same time that most states and the federal government impose severe restrictions on embryonic research that could potentially help cure innumerable diseases, in other states, such as California, embryos can be created from "donor" eggs and "donor" sperm—purchased by the clinic from donors with desirable traits (tall, thin, well educated)—for the explicit purpose of being sold to patients. "These are not donated embryos," explains Andrew Vorzimer, a California-based fertility lawyer, on his blog, in reference to the created embryos that are owned by the fertility clinic. "Rather, they are embryos created from donors hand-selected by California Conceptions. It is one step removed from a mail order catalog. The only difference is that the product being sold is nascent human life." Noting the large numbers of "unwanted human embryos in the United States," Vorzimer concludes that "donated embryos do not make for a very profitable business model."[15] But clients, having suffered years of infertility, praise the program, which offers three tries and a money-back guarantee, as well as success rates (self-reported) pushing 75 percent while eliminating potential uncertainty that could result from adoption. When asked by Dr. Ernest Zeringue, founder of California Conceptions, whether the practice was ethically acceptable, the ASRM said the ethics committee thought it would be premature to issue an opinion.[16]

The science and technology of fertility treatments will likely continue to outpace our society's ability to confront the legal and ethical challenges spawned by these advances. Techniques such as mitochondrial replacement therapy and gene editing raise a new generation of ethical and policy questions that undoubtedly will be handled in different ways around the globe, and throughout the United States.

On April 6, 2016, a healthy baby boy was born to Jordanian parents who had been trying to start a family for nearly twenty years in what has been described as a normal, trouble-free birth. The young Jordanian's conception, however, was far from run-of-the-mill. Born to a mother with Leigh syndrome, a severe neurological disorder that is passed on through the mother, the boy is the first to be born as a result of an innovative and controversial technology known as mitochondrial replacement therapy (MRT), or mitochondrial donation.

Mitochondria, known as the powerhouses or batteries of the human cell, sit outside a cell's nucleus and contain tiny quantities of DNA, provided solely by the mother. Their function is to provide the cell's energy, rather than conferring genetic traits; genes in the cell's nucleus, containing DNA from both mother and father, determine inherited characteristics such as appearance and intelligence.

Mutations in mitochondrial DNA can cause a wide variety of devastating conditions, which are guaranteed to be passed on to the next generation through the mother's DNA. A mother with Leigh syndrome caused by a mitochondrial mutation, therefore, would pass it on to her children, as this Jordanian mother had come to learn all too painfully, experiencing four miscarriages as well as the death of two children, one at eight months and one at six years old.

The couple eventually found their way to Dr. Zhang, of New Hope Fertility Center, and learned about MRT. The type of mitochondrial transfer he proposed, known as spindle nuclear transfer, enables doctors to create an embryo with the genetic material of three "biological parents" by taking the nucleus out of the mother's egg, which has unhealthy mitochondria, and injecting it into a donor egg (which has had its nucleus removed) that has healthy mitochondria. The mitochondrial DNA from the donor egg will comprise only 0.05 to 0.2 percent of the DNA of the resulting embryo.

Banned by Congress in the United States, Dr. Zhang and his team traveled with his Jordanian patients to Mexico, where there are no laws that prohibit the procedure, generating both praise and criticism. Supporters hailed the birth as a triumph for progressive medicine with the potential to both eliminate certain incurable genetic diseases and provide hope and relief to the families confronting the pain of mitochondrial disease. Critics called it irresponsible, arguing that not enough research had been done to know whether it was safe. Opponents also questioned the long-term implications of creating children with DNA from three parents; any daughters born would pass on this new "combined" DNA (known as germ modification) to their future offspring, the consequences of which are unknown. In the case of the Jordanian family, because the child is a boy, he is incapable of transferring the combined DNA to any future children, sidestepping the ethical question for now.

Ironically, the technique, which is not entirely new, was developed in the United States and then forced offshore due to regulation. The precursor to MRT, known as cytoplasmic transfer, was pioneered in the late 1990s by Dr. Jacques Cohen and his team at the Saint Barnabas Institute in New Jersey. Cytoplasm is a jellylike substance that surrounds the nucleus and contains mitochondria. Treating a patient who had been trying to have a baby for ten years, Dr. Cohen suspected that there was a chance that some structure in the cytoplasm didn't function optimally, and one of the major candidates was mitochondria. Dr. Cohen transferred a small amount of cytoplasm from a donor to his patient's egg and then fertilized the egg with her husband's sperm. Nine months later, long-awaited Alana was born. Sixteen more babies followed under Dr. Cohen's care. Others copied the technique, and Dr. Cohen estimates that some thirty to fifty babies were born as a result of cytoplasmic transfer. But in 2002, the FDA stepped in and asked clinics to stop doing the procedure, citing safety and ethical concerns, particularly the theoretical concern about genetic modification. Since then, the procedure has not been performed in the United Sates.

Despite subsequent efforts to reverse this stance by the National Academies of Science, Engineering and Medicine as well as the FDA as the science has evolved, Congress remains firm in upholding its ban of the procedure. Paradoxically, some critics as well as proponents would like to see the procedure brought onshore. Noting what he calls "problems with the study," in reference to Dr. Zhang's work on mitochondrial replacement therapy, Dr. Dieter Egli of Columbia University Medical Center believes that the FDA should be overseeing these procedures. "For a technique pioneered and developed in the US, it [would] be fitting to see the benefits to patients here as well," he wrote to NPR news. "Because of funding restrictions to the FDA, promising medical advances are forced to move elsewhere."[17]

The British Parliament in 2015 voted to allow mitochondrial donation, making the United Kingdom the first country in the world to permit IVF babies to be created using biological material from three different people in order to help prevent serious genetic diseases. The British law allows for a procedure known as pronuclear transfer, which involves fertilizing both the mother's egg and a donor egg with the father's sperm. Before the fertilized eggs start dividing into early-stage embryos, their nuclei are removed. The nucleus from the donor's fertilized egg is discarded and replaced by that from the mother's fertilized egg. While critics, like in the United States, opposed the technique on ethical grounds, supporters, highlighting the pain and difficulty of caring for a child with a devastating disease, promoted the lifesaving benefits of MRT and countered critics by pointing out that having a third person's DNA in your system is nothing new. Comparing the donation of mitochondria to his giving bone marrow to someone suffering from leukemia, Dr. Peter Braude, emeritus professor of obstetrics and gynecology at King's College London, pointed out that from the transplant onward, the recipient will have DNA from Dr. Braude: "You won't be related to me, you may be grateful to me, but you will have DNA from a third person circulating in your body."[18]

The first baby conceived as a result of pronuclear transfer was born to a previously infertile mother on January 5, 2017, in Kiev, Ukraine.[19] The mother, who did not suffer from mitochondrial disease, had tried unsuccessfully to have a baby for over a decade, with four failed IVF cycles.

Gene editing, while an entirely different technology from MRT, presents similar questions and challenges, particularly with respect to the ethics of altering the genetic line. In April 2015, a group of Chinese researchers sparked an international frenzy when they revealed that they had completed the world's first experiments in editing genes in a human embryo—a technique that could potentially help prevent or eliminate genetic diseases and birth defects. Using the cutting-edge technology of a new gene editor called CRISPR-Cas9, which allows researchers to easily make precise cuts in the DNA of an embryo, the Chinese team tried to correct a mutation that causes a blood disease.[20]

The Chinese were quickly joined by Britain and Sweden. The United Kingdom's Human Fertilisation and Embryology Authority (HFEA) in early 2016 approved research on editing the genomes of human embryos. Developmental biologist Dr. Kathy Niakan and her team at the Francis Crick Institute in London are editing genes in embryos that are active just after fertilization, and could potentially lead to treatments for infertility. After just seven days, the embryos will be destroyed. Dr. Fredrik Lanner of the Karolinska Institutet in Stockholm is similarly editing genes in viable human embryos with an eye to exploring early human development. Scientists speculate that there are more private groups out there doing this kind of work, but that they haven't opened up their labs to public scrutiny.[21]

In August 2017, gene editing was conducted for the first time in the United States. A team of researchers, led by Dr. Shoukhrat Mitalipov, a reproductive biology specialist at the Oregon Health & Science University, successfully used CRISPR-Cas9 technology to correct the MYBPC3 gene that causes hypertrophic cardiomyopathy, a potentially fatal heart condition. Although the research is in early stages and must overcome

regulatory and scientific hurdles prior to clinical use, researchers believe that in the future, this technique could be used in conjunction
with PGD to help fix mutations in embryos that would otherwise be
discarded. One of the biggest obstacles? The lack of federal funding for
embryonic research.

The US bans on federal funding are likely to drive evolving technologies such as mitochondrial replacement therapy and gene editing, like
most infertility research, to the private sector or overseas.[22] Dr. Mitalipov, for example, said that he would be willing to move his research to
the United Kingdom, if necessary.[23]

In 1974, Congress enacted a temporary moratorium on all federally
funded clinical research on embryos and embryonic tissue, including
research on IVF, infertility, and prenatal diagnosis, until national guidelines were established. Presumably sometime in the not-too-distant future. *Forty-four years later, that moratorium is still in place*, hampering not
only progress in combatting infertility, but also the potential development of lifesaving therapies for a wide range of diseases. In addition
to denying researchers much-needed funding and slowing scientific
progress, the moratorium also deprives privately funded research (and
therefore the public) of government oversight, which would, for example, verify that studies are carried out in an ethically acceptable way,
protecting infertile couples that may be vulnerable to exploitation or
ensuring that embryos are not used without consent or sold for profit.

With the rapid evolution of technology, how will doctors and lawmakers in the United States, which lacks comprehensive regulation of
even basic IVF and other fertility treatments more than thirty-five years
after their inception, be prepared to face questions raised by scientific
advances? The future is upon us, and our policy makers cannot ignore
it any longer.

Completing a book, it's a little like having a baby.

John le Carré

Epilogue

Watching our children grow and develop into the independent little people that they are—catching glimpses of Alexandra dancing, and William building, and the two of them engaging in their own in-depth conversations—I sometimes find myself lost in thought, marveling at the very fact that they *exist*. I always knew how much I wanted them, but I never anticipated how much joy they would bring into our lives. Yet for every surge of joy, I know that there is another woman or man or couple out there who has not enjoyed such success, who has given up or is still trying—and I know we could be doing so much more to help them get there.

When I reflect on my long journey, on the many years of desperately wanting and trying, and finally ultimately succeeding against the odds to have our children, I'm aware of my own personal process of evolution—of how I changed irreversibly. Somewhere along the way, I transformed from a woman who was afraid of needles and resisted shots with all my might to a fearless warrior who mixed potions, loaded syringes, and casually injected myself while talking to clients on speakerphone, in the ladies' room in restaurants and nightclubs, and even once in the Moroccan desert on Christmas Eve. I morphed from a patient who didn't believe I needed IVF to a client perpetually cycling through it, all in the effort to produce our two scientific miracles.

By the time our kids are old enough to read and understand the story of their conception, I am guessing that it will not be as unusual to contemplate that there were at least three—but closer actually to a dozen—people involved in bringing them into the world, rather than just the prince and princess they are accustomed to seeing in modern media. That there was Mom and Dad; and Catherine, our practically perfect surrogate; as well as the fertility specialists, embryologists, anesthesiologists, ultrasound technicians, acupuncturists, nurses, aides, midwives, and an alchemist. Not to mention those who helped us along the way down the paths not ultimately taken: the adoption specialists, home study social worker, other adoptive parents, and potential egg donors from around the world.

I imagine that their world will look quite different.

The future that I envision for our children is one in which these crucial gaps are closed. A world in which infertility treatment is viewed as a medical problem and covered by mainstream insurance policies. Where treatment is within reach financially for all who need and desire it. Where donors and surrogates are compensated fairly yet not astronomically.

A world in which patients are informed consumers of their treatment, aware of options and differing approaches. Where drugs are dispensed in a more incremental approach, rather than the kitchen-sink approach often used in America today. Where hormones are prescribed in the lowest effective dosages, both saving money and protecting the health of consumers.

A world in which federal funding is available to support research that advances scientific knowledge and informs both medical treatment and the establishment of sensible regulations.

I look at Alexandra and William and hope that they will live in such a world. It doesn't seem too much to wish for, given that they already live in a world that was able to give them the miracle of life.

Afterword

BY DR. JOEL BATZOFIN,
MD, FACOG, Medical Director,
New York Fertility Services, Manhattan, New York

*A*nyone who has struggled with infertility understands at a fundamental level just how all-consuming this problem can be. Not infrequently, a couple transitions from being concerned about the efficacy of a particular form of contraception to the realization that they have a problem conceiving. It takes courage to seek help for such an intimate aspect of one's life. Sadly, in many cases, care can be the start of a long, challenging, and expensive journey through a maze of diagnostic tests and treatments. Some 15 to 20 percent of couples seeking to start or enlarge their family are affected by infertility.

As a consequence of her own years-long struggle with infertility, Elizabeth Katkin not only brings a wealth of knowledge and personal experience but also provides readers with useful insights she learned on her long, complex, transcontinental journey.

Katkin has lived, worked, and sought fertility treatments in different cities, countries, and continents. From her native United States to London, Dubai, and Russia, Katkin's journey transformed her "from an ardent believer in following doctors' orders to an active advocate" for herself. Readers of this book have learned about the complexities and challenges associated with a diagnosis of infertility. They have also learned about the importance of staying committed to the cause and about never giving up hope for solutions. Her story is a testament that no couples or individuals should remain involuntarily childless.

Katkin suffered infertility and multiple miscarriages as a consequence of polycystic ovarian syndrome, aneuploidy, as well as immune-related infertility. Any one of these complex problems can be challenging enough; together they at times may seem insurmountable. Fortunately, through the marvels of modern medicine, as well as her own commitment and the expertise of her doctors, Katkin and her husband are now the parents of two healthy children. Having been involved in this quest as a provider of care for some of the journey, I can attest to the persistence and unwavering devotion to the project that Elizabeth and her husband, Richard, demonstrated.

Through her personal story, hopefully Katkin has inspired readers to recognize that there is not a "one size fits all" approach to treatment. She challenges several conventional dogmas. Her story forces even the most experienced practitioner to question some of his or her own beliefs and practices. Furthermore, through the complex ethical, philosophical, and moral realities, readers pause and evaluate where they stand on some of the most pressing issues involved in reproductive medicine.

Recognizing that the practice of reproductive medicine is both a business as well as a treatment involving sophisticated high-tech solutions to complex medical problems, Katkin helps the reader to understand aspects of their care, which may not initially be readily apparent. She understands how vulnerable patients are, and she cautions them against falling into traps they may later regret. She encourages patients to recognize themselves as consumers and to undertake the necessary due diligence. Her legal expertise raises intelligent and provocative questions regarding regulatory aspects of the field. She addresses challenging concepts such as mitochondrial replacement therapy (so-called three-parent babies) and gene editing; disposal of unused embryos; custodial aspects of frozen embryos; and the sale of frozen embryos.

Conceivability is an extremely informative and well-researched book. Besides giving hope to anyone confronting this challenging disease called infertility, it is also a story of optimism and triumph. Katkin describes how she hopes her children will live in a world where patients avail themselves of state-of-the-art treatments, delivered safely, ethically, legally, and successfully anywhere they live in the world.

Any health-care provider involved in reproductive medicine, and any patient confronting this disease, will be happy they invested the time to read *Conceivability*. Readers are rewarded with finding answers to some vexing questions, as explained by a true fertility warrior, who has demonstrated amazing tenacity and persistence in search of her dreams.

Acknowledgments

Although it is long established that brevity is the soul of wit, I am afraid that in this case, I am simply unable to oblige, for there are far too many good souls to whom I am indebted.

This book started out as a thought on the beaches of Dubai in the months before William arrived, and evolved through conversations over coffee, hummus, and wine, through fits and starts, as the days turned into years. It was nurtured at the beginning and again at the end, both personally and professionally, by my good friend (very conveniently a book editor) Liza Darnton, who insisted from the beginning that I needed to write a Big Book, not just a memoir. *Conceivability* may never have emerged beyond my dreams, however, if I hadn't been introduced to my very talented agent, Gillian MacKenzie, who saw the potential in this project and helped me to develop and refine my vision for the book. Thank you, Gillian.

I am so very grateful for Marysue Rucci, who took a bet on me, sharing my enthusiasm for bringing this information into the world, and helping me to shape an enormous, disparate mass of material into a relatable, digestible whole. Her intelligent questions and thoughtful reads pushed me to dig deeper. Many thanks as well to the marvelous team at Simon & Schuster, who all played key roles in launching *Conceivability*: Zachary Knoll, Christine Masters, Erica Ferguson, Amanda Lang, Lauren Carsley, and Dana Trocker.

Of course, there would be no book if there were no babies, and for that, I must thank my impressive, and extensive, medical team. First and foremost, Dr. Joel Batzofin, a wonderful doctor and now friend, treated us with so much care and respect, explaining every treatment each step of the way, and was never rushed for time. Without him, and Teresa and Kayee and the rest of his team, we would not have Alexandra. On the other side of the world, Dr. Oxana Bykovskaya and her team at AltraVita opened my eyes to the possibility of a second child, and delivered on that promise, bringing William into our lives. Mr. Jeffrey Braithwaite, assisted by his wife and practice manager, Jane, and nurse Maria, treated us with tender, loving, and thoughtful care every step of the way, through uncountable exams and ultrasounds in support of our attempts, numerous miscarriages, and ultimately, two births.

And we had so much additional help from caring medical professionals along the way: Dr. Preston Sacks in DC; Drs. Yau Thum and Marie Wren at the Lister in London; Dr. Rachel Ashby at Brigham and Women's in Massachusetts; Dr. Nataliya Petrova at the Cooper Health Clinic in Dubai; Dr. George Lewin at Southampton Medical Centre; the dedicated and caring nurses and midwives at the Maternity Unit at Ormskirk and District General Hospital who cared for all of us at the births of both Alexandra and William; and Dr. Victoria Muir of Belgrave Medical Centre and the kind staff of her baby clinic, who were always there for our family, before, during, and after the arrival of our beloved children. Special thanks as well to my outstanding acupuncturists and practitioners of traditional Chinese medicine: Dr. Mengda Shu in DC, who made me believe; Dr. Xiao-Ping Zhai of the Zhai Clinic in London; and the ever-ebullient Louisa Gordon, who saw me through, well, a lot. We are also eternally grateful to the amazing Ann Haigh, who skillfully and cheerfully steered us not only through the British parental order system but also through the unexpected complexity of obtaining William's US passport.

I am also convinced that there would be neither book nor babies without the massive, unending support of my incredible family and friends who sustained me through years of infertility and miscarriage. While our network of friends spans several countries, I was fortunate to have a core group of amazing women in London who, with love, brainpower, care, and humor, saw me through my darkest days: Julie Lasso, Susan Namkung, Irene Chang, Kathryn Peterson, Sharon Benning, Trisha Johnson, Trish Thomas, Aleksandra Dochnal. How can I ever thank you? My dear friend Kathy Economy, from the beaches of Koh Samui to the hospital halls of the Brigham, has always had my back, and for this I am very grateful. Rod Baker, my friend and colleague, kindly led us through the English legal system, while other members of my Hogan "family"—Steve Robinson, Jeff Hurlburt, John Basnage, Mike Cheroutes, George Hagerty, Sean Harrison, Sharon Gray Edwards, Danielle Wood—somehow kept me together at work. Rustam Aksenenko and Svetlana Cheshinskaya supported our attempts and explorations from IVF to immunology to Russian adoption, from London to Geneva to Frankfurt to Moscow; no favor was too big or small. Jeffrey Costello and Olga Skorik counseled, housed, fed, translated for, transported, and ultimately celebrated with us; it's a joy to see our Sashas and their younger brothers play together.

And then there are the friends that saw me through my "new" baby project: this book. Brandt Goldstein, a writer and lifelong friend, initiated me into the world of nonfiction writing, providing all-important guidance and feedback. John Pollack was at the ready with humor, advice, and a helping hand. Brad Meltzer and Cori Flam were a source of constant support and enthusiasm, not only willing but also seeking out ways to assist me. Ulcca Joshi Hansen brainstormed and commiserated with me. Noelle Salmi has shared her great ideas with me for more than twenty-five years. The members of my now sadly defunct writing group—Carrie Bach, Diana Dresser, Liz and Sue Tencate—got me started on the daunting task. Merry Logan assisted in shaping my very first proposal, while my walks and talks with Rachel Moskovich helped me find my way when I was lost. Nicole Jacques always had a glass of wine and good cheer when I needed it most. And the wonderful talent of Emily Rapp Black and the members of her Lighthouse Writers Workshop Lit Fest gave me a boost when I needed it most, their critical feedback and creative stimulation rallying me toward the finish line.

I owe an enormous debt of gratitude to the many patients I met and interviewed for this project. Your stories moved me, awed me, and inspired me to write a book that might help others avoid some of your—our—pain. For privacy reasons, I won't name you, but you all know who you are. I am honored that you chose to share your very personal journeys with me.

Many heartfelt thanks as well to the experts who contributed to my understanding of a very complex field. Jane Gregorie of Acupuncture Denver is a Renaissance woman—writer, practitioner, patient, connector, editor, mother—who provided invaluable aid. Dr. Neil Box generously helped me understand some of the underlying genetics concepts. Dr. Lori Bernstein shared her personal journey and groundbreaking research with me. Dr. Joan Manheimer helped illuminate the many painful feelings men and women confronting infertility experience. I am extremely grateful to the organizers of the 2016 ART World Congress in New York (Dr. John Zhang, Dr. Yanping Kuang, and Dr. Keiichi Kato) and the 24th World Congress on Controversies in Obstetrics, Gynecology & Infertility in Amsterdam (Dr. Zion Ben Rafael, Dr. Bart C.J.M. Fauser, and Dr. Rene Frydman) for allowing me access as an observer. The knowledge I gained was invaluable, and I would particularly like to thank the generous specialists who helped me to expand my understanding: Dr. Mark Hughes, Dr. Santiago Munné, Dr. Jacques Cohen, and Dr. Simon Fishel.

As for Catherine Hardy, there are no words. With style, grace, humility, kindness, and compassion, Catherine gave us the most extraordinary gift a person can give. How does one thank someone for, literally, the gift of life? I am forever not only grateful but also genuinely happy that Catherine entered our lives, and brought along her beautiful family: her daughter, Eden; mother, Denise; grandmother, Jess; and sisters, Jac and Nic. It has been the greatest pleasure watching Catherine and Eden blossom as they achieve their own dreams.

And finally, of course, last only in paragraph order, is my family. If I must trace the origins of my stubborn, relentless quest to have children, I must go back to the very beginning. I was blessed to grow up bathed in the unconditional love of a truly wonderful family. Not only my fantastic parents and brother, Ken, but also our grandparents, aunts and uncles, so many wonderful cousins; my cousin Beth, like a sister to me, has been my greatest cheerleader. And then the next generation arrived—my niece and nephew, and cousins' children—and watching them grow up, I knew I wanted that too. My devoted parents, Wendy and Edward, who have supported me wholeheartedly in all of my adventures, truly outdid themselves here. My mother tirelessly read every draft, served as an unpaid research assistant, connected me with women with stories to tell, entertained her grandchildren when I had deadlines, and throughout it all, prodded me to take care of myself, reminding me that I was her baby.

Richard is my rock, my soul mate, my partner. Little did he know when we said those vows many moons ago what "for better or worse" would encompass. Yet through years of failed attempts, heartbreaking miscarriages, unyielding schedules, he never wavered. He just loved me; propped me up when I was down; helped me navigate our path toward our children. I am so grateful that our challenges drew us ever closer together, and that our success allowed me to add fantastic father to his job description. Alexandra and William, our two modern miracles, I thank for their joy, love, and patience with Mommy's seemingly never-ending work. Kids, it's really done this time.

Notes

Introduction

1. Nicholas Bakaler, "U.S. Fertility Rate Reaches a Record Low," *New York Times*, July 3, 2017.

2. According to the National Survey of Family Growth (NSFG), from 2011 to 2015, 12.1 percent of all women, or approximately 7.3 million women, experienced problems getting pregnant or carrying a baby to term and 14.2 percent of all married women in that period were categorized as infertile, down from 16.2 percent in 2002. See Key Statistics from National Survey of Family Growth at https://www.cdc.gov/nchs/nsfg/key_statistics/i .htm#infertility, accessed December 10, 2017. See also a CDC Infertility White Paper entitled "A Public Health Focus on Infertility Prevention, Detection, and Management" at https://www.cdc.gov/reproductivehealth /infertility/whitepaper-pg1.htm.

3. Ibid. Nearly 2 percent of women of childbearing age had medical visits in a twelve-month period ending in 2002. See A. Chandra, G. M. Martinez, W. D. Mosher, et al., "Fertility, Family Planning, and Reproductive Health of U.S. Women: Data from the 2002 National Survey of Family Growth," National Center for Health Statistics, *Vital and Health Statistics* 23, no. 25 (December 2005): 1–160.

According to the NSFG, from 2001 to 2015, 12 percent of women aged fifteen to forty-four, or 7.3 million women, and 17 percent of women aged twenty-five to forty-four (6.9 million women) in the United States had received infertility services. See A. Chandra, C. E. Copen, and E. H. Stephen, "Infertility Service Use in the United States: Data from the National Survey of Family Growth, 1928–2010," Centers for Disease Control and Prevention, US Department of Health and Human Services, National Health Statistics Reports, no. 73 (January 22, 2014).

Chapter 1

1. For a detailed description of the evolution of the use of hormones, see Debora L. Spar, *The Baby Business* (Cambridge, MA: Harvard Business Review Press, 2006), 18–21.

2. Quoted in Barbara Seaman, "Is This Any Way to Have a Baby?," *O, The Oprah Magazine*, February 2004. Available online, with the permission of the author, on *Evidence-Based Perspectives on Hot Women's Health Issues*, https:// gilliansanson.wordpress.com/2004/02/07/is-this-any-way-to-have-a -baby-by-barbara-seaman/.

3. Shady Grove Fertility, "Clomid for Infertility: What You Need to Know," July 13, 2016, https://www.shadygrovefertility.com/blog/treatments -and-success/clomid-for-infertility/.

4. Andrea Manzi-Davies, "Helena Bonham Carter: 'I would have tried anything, even IVF,'" *The Telegraph*, October 15, 2007, https://www .telegraph.co.uk/women/womens-health/3351623/Helena-Bonham -Carter-I-would-have-tried-anything-even-IVF.html.

5. According to Christine Lee, MD, who also holds a PhD in developmental biology and an MS in biomolecular organization and serves as lab director of ConceiveEasy, the incidence of twins is approximately 8 to 10 percent for clomiphene pregnancies. Christine Lee, "What are the Chances of Having Twins with Clomid?", February 19, 2014, https://www.conceiveeasy .com/get-pregnant/what-are-the-chances-of-having-twins-with-clomid -2/. The ASRM advises patients that of women who achieve pregnancy with clomiphene citrate, approximately 5 to 12 percent bear twins. See American Society for Reproductive Medicine, *Multiple Pregnancy and Birth: Twins, Triplets, and High-order Multiples: A Guide for Patients*, 2012, http://www

.reproductivefacts.org/news-and-publications/patient-fact-sheets-and
-booklets/fact-sheets-and-info-booklets/multiple-pregnancy-and-birth
-twins-triplets-and-high-order-multiples-booklet/.

6. Irene Moy and Geraldine Ekpo, "Clomiphene Citrate Use for Ovulation Induction: When, Why, and How?," *Contemporary OB/GYN*, April 1,
2011, http://contemporaryobgyn.modernmedicine.com/contemporary
-obgyn/news/clinical/clinical-pharmacology/clomiphene-citrate
-use-ovulation-induction-wh?page=full. Although the cause of ovarian hyperstimulation syndrome (OHSS) is not fully understood, having a high
level of human chorionic gonadotropin (HCG) introduced into a woman's
system had been established to play a role. While mild to moderate OHSS
is more common and usually goes away after about a week, approximately
1 to 2 percent of women undergoing ovarian stimulation develop a severe
form of OHSS, which can be life-threatening. Injectable fertility medications are more likely to cause OHSS than Clomid. See Mayo Clinic, "Ovarian Hyperstimulation Syndrome," accessed December 10, 2017, http://
www.mayoclinic.org/diseases-conditions/ovarian-hyperstimulation-syn
drome-ohss/symptoms-causes/dxc-20263586.

7. Mark Fainaru-Wada and Lance Williams, "Giambi admitted taking steroids," *SFGate*, December 2, 2004, https://www.sfgate.com/sports/ar
ticle/Giambi-admitted-taking-steroids-2631890.php.

8. Moy and Ekpo, "Clomiphene Citrate Use," and Shady Grove Fertility, "Clomid for Infertility."

9. Ibid.

10. E. Hughes, J. Brown, J. J. Collins, and P. Vanderkerchove, "Clomiphene
Citrate for Unexplained Subfertility in Women," *Cochrane Database of Systematic Reviews*, no.1 (January 20, 2010): article ID CD000057.

11. Rotterdam ESHRE/ASRM-Sponsored PCOS Consensus Workshop
Group, "Revised 2003 Consensus on Diagnostic Criteria and Long-term
Health Risks Related to Polycystic Ovary Syndrome," *Fertility and Sterility*
81, no. 1 (January 2004):19–25.

12. American Congress of Obstetricians and Gynecologists (ACOG) Committee on Practice Bulletins—Gynecology, "ACOG Practice Bulletin
No. 108: Polycystic Ovary Syndrome," *Obstetrics & Gynecology 114*, no. 4
(October 2009): 936–49. Reaffirmed 2015, https://www.acog.org/Re
sources-And-Publications/Practice-Bulletins-List.

13. National Institutes of Health, "New Treatment Increases Pregnancy Rate for Women with Infertility Disorder," news release, July 9, 2014, https://www.nih.gov/news-events/news-releases/new-treatment-increases-pregnancy-rate-women-infertility-disorder. R. F. Casper and M. F. Mitwally, "Review: Aromatase Inhibitors for Ovulation Induction," *Journal of Clinical Endocrinology and Metabolism* 91, no. 3 (March 2006): 760–71.

14. NIH, "New Treatment." The study, which had fifty-seven collaborators, was conducted by the Reproductive Medicine Network of NIH's Eunice Kennedy Shriver National Institute of Child Health and Human Development (NICHD). R. S. Legro, R. G. Brzyski, M. P. Diamond, et al., "Letrozole versus Clomiphene for Infertility in the Polycystic Ovary Syndrome. *New England Journal of Medicine* 371 (2014): 119–29.

15. Ibid. See also Shirley S. Wang, "Study Shows Letrozole's Efficacy in Boosting Pregnancy Chances," *Wall Street Journal*, July 9, 2014, https://www.wsj.com/articles/study-shows-letrozoles-efficacy-in-boosting-pregnancy-chances-1404939604.

16. NIH, "New Treatment."

Chapter 2

1. Richard Sherbahn, "Anti-Mullerian Hormone Testing of Ovarian Reserve," Advanced Fertility Center of Chicago, accessed December 10, 2017, http://www.advancedfertility.com/amh-fertility-test.htm.

2. See "What Is anti-Müllerian Hormone (AMH)?" in Shady Grove Fertility, "Fertility Facts: Anti-Müllerian Hormone (AMH) Can Help Predict Your Ovarian Reserve," June 23, 2017, https://www.shadygrovefertility.com/blog/diagnosing-infertility/fertility-facts-anti-mullerian-hormone-amh-can-help-predict-your-ovarian-reserve/.

3. Sherbahn, "Anti-Mullerian Hormone Testing."

Chapter 3

1. Quoted in Colette Bouchez, "The Ancient Art of Infertility Treatment," WebMD Feature, October 13, 2003, https://www.webmd.com/infertility-and-reproduction/features/ancient-art-of-infertility-treatment#1.

2. A study in Tel Aviv found that acupuncture and herbs used in conjunction

with IUI increased the IUI success rate from 39.4 percent to 65.5 percent. K. Sela, O. Lehavi, A. Buchan, et al., "Acupuncture and Chinese Herbal Treatment for Women Undergoing Intrauterine Insemination," *European Journal of Integrative Medicine* 3, no. 2 (June 2011): e77–81.

A meta-analysis of seven trials found that acupuncture treatments on the same day as embryo transfer increased the odds of clinical pregnancy by 65 percent. E. Manheimer, G. Zhang, L. Udoff, et al., "Effects of Acupuncture on Rates of Pregnancy and Live Birth Among Women Undergoing In Vitro Fertilization: Systematic Review and Meta-analysis," *BMJ* 336, no. 7,643 (March 8, 2008): 545–49. See also Serena Gordon, "Acupuncture May Boost Pregnancy Success Rates," *U.S. News & World Report*, January 27, 2012, online edition, https://health.usnews.com/health-news/family -health/womens-health/articles/2012/01/27/acupuncture-may-boost -pregnancy-success-rates.

3. See Randine Lewis, *The Infertility Cure: The Ancient Chinese Wellness Program for Getting Pregnant and Having Healthy Babies*, reprint ed. (Boston: Little, Brown, 2005); Gordon, "Acupuncture May Boost"; Pacific College of Oriental Medicine, "How Does Acupuncture for Fertility Work? Increase Chance of Conception without Side Effects," updated September 4, 2017, http://www.pacificcollege.edu/news/blog/2015/04/17/how-does-acu puncture-fertility-work-increase-chance-conception-without-side.

4. Jane Gregorie, interview with the author, March 22, 2016.

5. L. E. Hullender Rubin, M. S. Opsahl, K. E. Wiemer, et al., "Impact of Whole Systems Traditional Chinese Medicine on In Vitro Fertilization Outcomes," *Reproductive BioMedicine Online* 30, no. 6 (June 2015): 602–12. See also Lewis, *Infertility Cure*.

6. The American Board of Oriental and Reproductive Medicine (ABORM) was founded to establish and maintain high standards among practitioners; as a result, members submit to a voluntary certification process. ABORM maintains an extensive database of certified specialists on their website (www.aborm.org), which extends far beyond US borders, not only to Canada but also to Switzerland, Australia, and New Zealand as well.

7. Randine Lewis, "The High FSH Craze," http://fertilefoods.com/the-high -fsh-craze/.

8. Jane Gregorie, interview with the author, March 22, 2016.

9. Elizabeth Stener-Victorin conducted breakthrough studies on reducing

hypertension in the uterine artery. E. Stener-Victorin, U. Waldenström, S. A. Andersson, and M. Wikland, " Reduction of Blood Flow Impedance in the Uterine Arteries of Infertile Women with Electro-acupuncture," *Human Reproduction* 11, no. 6 (June 1996): 1314–17.

10. J. Johansson and E. Stener-Victorin, "Polycystic Ovary Syndrome: Effect and Mechanisms of Acupuncture for Ovulation Induction," *Evidence-Based Complementary and Alternative Medicine* 2013 (2013): 16 pages, article ID 762615.

11. Gordon, "Acupuncture May Boost."

12. P. C. Magarelli, D. K. Cridennda, and M. Cohen, "Changes in Serum Cortisol and Prolactin Associated with Acupuncture During Controlled Ovarian Hyperstimulation in Women Undergoing In Vitro Fertilization–Embryo Transfer Treatment," *Fertility and Sterility* 92, no. 6 (December 2009): 1870–9.

13. See, for example, J. Pei, E. Strehler, U. Noss, et al., "Quantitative Evaluation of Spermatozoa Ultrastructure After Acupuncture Treatment for Idiopathic Male Fertility," *Fertility and Sterility* 84, no. 1 (July 2005): 141–47.

14. Elizabeth Palermo, "What Is Acupuncture?" *LiveScience*, June 21, 2017, https://www.livescience.com/29494-acupuncture.html.

15. Quoted in Rachel Gurevich, "How Does Acupuncture Help Fertility? Ancient and Modern Theories on Why Acupuncture May Improve Fertility," *Verywell*, updated December 1, 2016, https://www.verywell.com/how-does-acupuncture-help-fertility-1959899.

16. Palermo, "What Is Acupuncture?"

17. Dr. Chang also advocates that acupuncture appears to have a neuroendocrine effect, strengthening a three-way axis between the hypothalamus and the pituitary glands (two areas of the brain involved with hormone production) and the ovaries, which ultimately impacts egg production and possibly ovulation.

18. Hua Liu, Jian-Yang Xu, Lin Li, et al., "fMRI Evidence of Acupoints Specificity in Two Adjacent Acupoints," *Evidence-Based Complementary and Alternative Medicine* 2013 (2013): 5 pages, article ID 932581.

19. Sela et al., "Acupuncture and Chinese Herbal Treatment."

20. Pei et al., "Quantitative Evaluation."

21. G. Franconi, L. Manni, L. Aloe, et al., "Acupuncture in Clinical and Experimental Reproductive Medicine: A Review," *Journal of Endocrinological Investigation* 34, no. 4 (April 2011): 307–11.

22. Ibid. Also, in 2002, a group of German researchers discovered that adding acupuncture to the traditional IVF treatment protocols substantially increased pregnancy success, finding that nearly half of women receiving just two twenty-five-minute sessions of acupuncture, one prior to having the fertilized embryos transferred into their uteri, and one directly afterward, had success getting pregnant, compared to just over a quarter of those who received no acupuncture treatments. W. E. Paulus, M. Zhang, E. Strehler, et al., "Influence of Acupuncture on the Pregnancy Rate in Patients Who Undergo Assisted Reproduction Therapy," *Fertility and Sterility* 77, no. 4 (April 2002): 721–24; S. Dieterle, G. Ying, W. Hatzmann, and A. Neuer, "Effect of Acupuncture on the Outcome of In Vitro Fertilization and Intracytoplasmic Sperm Injection: A Randomized, Prospective, Controlled Clinical Study," *Fertility and Sterility* 85, no. 5 (May 2006): 1347–51.

    Yet the research is not entirely clear. Although a meta-analysis of seven trials found that acupuncture treatments on the same day as embryo transfer increased the odds of clinical pregnancy by 65 percent (Manheimer et al., "Effects of Acupuncture"), later trials indicated that similar protocols of acupuncture treatments on the day of embryo transfer did not improve pregnancy rates compared with control groups. Y. C. Cheong, S. Dix, E. Hung Yu Ng, et al., "Acupuncture and Assisted Reproductive Technology," *Cochrane Database of Systematic Reviews*, no. 7 (July 26, 2013): article ID CD006920. A small American study that duplicated the German methodology did not find any improvement in pregnancy rates with acupuncture.

23. Quoted in Gordon, "Acupuncture May Boost."

24. For instance, a group of clinicians and researchers in Oregon designed the first comprehensive study to compare the results of IVF cycles carried out in conjunction with whole-systems TCM against the IVF results of cycles paired with just two acupuncture treatments on the day of embryo transfer and cycles that involved only the usual IVF care without any TCM intervention. Hullender Rubin et al., "Impact of Whole Systems." Their findings that an increased number of acupuncture treatments led to greater pregnancy and live birth outcomes echo the results of earlier studies on specific outcomes resulting from repetitive acupuncture sessions. For example, blood flow to the uterus was found to improve with eight electroacupuncture sessions (Stener-Victorin et al., "Reduction of Blood Flow"), serum cortisol

and prolactin were increased with a corresponding increase in IVF out-comes after nine electroacupuncture sessions (Magarelli et al., "Changes in Serum Cortisol"), and women with polycystic ovaries experienced im-proved menstrual regularity and reduced androgen levels after fourteen electro-acupuncture treatments (E. Jedel, F. Labrie, A. Oden, et al., "Im-pact of Electro-acupuncture and Physical Exercise on Hyperandrogenism and Oligo/Amenorrhea in Women with Polycystic Ovary Syndrome: A Randomized Controlled Trial," *American Journal of Physiology-Endocrinology and Metabolism* 300, no. 1 (January 2011): e37–45.

Chapter 4

1. For further information on toxoplasmosis and its potential effects on preg-nancy, see the CDC, Parasites-Toxoplasmosis (Toxoplasma infection) at https://www.cdc.gov/parasites/toxoplasmosis/gen_info/pregnant.html.
2. One study found the frequency of chromosomal abnormalities to be 69.4 percent. M. Ohno, T. Maeda, and A. Matsunobu, "A Cytogenetic Study of Spontaneous Abortions with Direct Analysis of Chorionic Villi," *Obstetrics & Gynecology* 77, no. 3 (March 1991): 394–98. Another study found that 70 to 90 percent of miscarriages occur due to chromosomal abnormalities. See IVF1, "Miscarriage History Raises Risk for Baby Chro-mosome Abnormalities," July 30, 2008, http://www.ivf1.com/miscar riage-risk/. For a more detailed discussion of the role of chromosomal abnormalities in miscarriage, please see chapter 8 and its notes.

Chapter 5

1. A typical round of IUI in the United States costs anywhere from $500 to $1,000 (up to $2,500 to $4,000, with medications and ultrasound moni-toring); expensive, but a drop in the bucket when compared to $12,000 to $25,000 for an IVF cycle.

Chapter 6

1. "What people worry about is that this is the first step on the road to Gattaca [referring to gender selection]," said Dr. Matt Wynia, the director of the

University of Colorado Center for Bioethics and Humanities. "Letting parents choose the height, eye color, IQ, etc. When you start thinking about those things being very expensive, you can imagine some future world in which only the wealthy can have a healthy, tall baby made to order," quoted in Jaclyn Allen, "Boy or Girl? More and More Colorado Parents Are Choosing Their Baby's Gender," Denver Channel, updated May 13, 2017, http://www.thedenverchannel.com/money/science-and-tech/boy-or-girl-more-and-more-colorado-parents-are-chosing-their-babys-gender. See also "Chrissy Teigen and John Legend Already Know the Gender of Their Second Baby—and Here's How," *Vogue*, November 21, 2017, https://www.vogue.com/article/chrissy-teigen-ivf-gender-selection-controversy-explained; and M. L. McGowan, and R. R. Sharp, "Justice in the Context of Family Balancing," *Science, Technology & Human Values* 38, no. 2 (March 1, 2013): article ID 10.1177/0162243912469412.

2. Margot Peppers, "The Rise of 'Social' Surrogacy: The Women Choosing Not to Carry Their Own Babies for Fear of Hurting Their Careers or Ruining Their Bodies, *Daily Mail* (UK), April 16, 2014, http://www.dailymail.co.uk/femail/article-2606101/the-rise-social-surrogacy-the-women-choosing-not-carry-babies-fear-hurting-careers-ruining-bodies.html#ixzz4t4OcD1ca. See also Sarah Elizabeth Richards, "Should a Woman Be Allowed to Hire a Surrogate Because She Fears Pregnancy Will Hurt Her Career?," *Elle*, April 17, 2014, http://www.elle.com/life-love/a14424/birth-rights/.

3. Critics fear the successful birth of a baby with three genetic parents, in a procedure performed to eliminate the possibility of passing on Leigh syndrome, an inherited genetic disorder, "could open the door to the creation of so-called designer babies." Rob Stein, "New York Fertility Doctor Says He Created Baby With 3 Genetic Parents," *All Things Considered*, NPR News, September 27, 2016, http://www.npr.org/sections/thetwo-way/2016/09/27/495668299/new-york-fertility-doctor-says-he-created-baby-with-3-genetic-parents.

4. Olivia Blair, "Chrissy Teigen Defends Selecting Gender of Her Baby During IVF After Backlash," *The Independent* (UK), February 24, 2016, http://www.independent.co.uk/news/people/chrissy-teigen-john-legend-baby-ivf-a6893621.html.

5. Interestingly, although many women I have spoken with shared this feeling, it is certainly not universal. Diana felt that the hardest part was getting

herself and her husband to a fertility clinic; she was relieved to just follow their instructions. Paula, on the other hand, had quite a different reaction to her first visit to a nationally recognized fertility specialist. "It was just a load of BS," she told me, still indignant years later, recalling her response to the diagnosis and advice she received. "I decided I was just going to wait and see what happened."

6. The first baby conceived with IVF using preimplantation genetic testing was born in 1990, and the technology has progressed dramatically in the last ten to fifteen years. For a more detailed discussion of the evolution of preimplantation genetic testing, see chapter 7, and Jason Franasiak and Richard T. Scott Jr., "A Brief History of Preimplantation Genetic Diagnosis and Preimplantation Genetic Screening," Virtual Academy of Genetics, http://www.ivf-worldwide.com/cogen/oep/pgd-pgs/history-of-pgd-and-pgs.html.

7. I had thought at the time that the Puregon contained synthetic FSH but have since learned that the solution for injection contains the active substance follitropin beta, produced by genetic engineering of a Chinese hamster ovary (CHO) cell line. See http://www.medicines.org.uk/emc/medicine/15946.

8. Also known as Pregnyl, Ovidrel, Novarel and others, all brand names for human chorionic gonadotropin (HCG).

9. Anna Magee, "Why Are So Many British Women Travelling Abroad for Fertility Treatment?," *The Telegraph* (UK), March 28, 2015, http://www.telegraph.co.uk/women/mother-tongue/11482483/fertility-treatment-why-british-women-are-travelling-abroad.html. M. Rezazadeh Valojerdi, P. Eftekhari-Yazdi, L. Karimian, et al., "Vitrification Versus Slow Freezing Gives Excellent Survival, Post Warming Embryo Morphology and Pregnancy Outcomes for Human Cleaved Embryos," *Journal of Assisted Reproduction and Genetics* 26, no. 6 (June 2009), 347–54.

Chapter 7

1. I injected 250 IUs of Puregon daily, up from 150 IUs.

2. At the time, Dr. Ashby referred to it as preimplantation genetic diagnosis (PGD) a more common term for both types of technology in 2004. As the technology has evolved, the terminology has correspondingly become more specific, and the type of genetic testing she was referring to is

now known as PGS. In order to avoid confusion, I refer to PGS, here and throughout, as it is generally used in 2017. A more detailed discussion of PGS and PGD can be found later in this chapter in the section entitled "Preimplantation Genetic Diagnosis (PGD) and Screening (PGS)".

3. For this cycle, I was prescribed Puregon, a form of FSH, plus Menopur, synthetic FSH combined with LH, as opposed to just FSH.

4. Viagra has been shown to increase the thickness of the uterine lining by increasing blood flow and estrogen delivery to the lining. See Geoffrey Sher, "Viagra as a Treatment to Thicken Uterine Lining," April 11, 2016, http://drgeoffreysherivf.com/viagra-treatment-thicken-uterine-lining/; R. D. Firouzabadi, R. Davar, F. Hojjat, and M. Mahdavi, "Effect of sildenafil citrate on endometrial preparation and outcome of frozen-thawed embryo transfer cycles: a randomized clinical trial," *Iranian Journal of Reproductive Medicine* 11, no. 2 (February 2013): 151–58.

5. Dr. Gillian Lockwood, the medical director of Midland Fertility Services, quoted in Magee, "British Women Travelling."

6. FertilityIQ, "Finding an IVF Doctor Is Total Hell," accessed December 11, 2017, https://www.fertilityiq.com/fertilityiq-data-and-notes/finding-an -ivf-doctor-is-total-hell.

7. Dr. Laura Rienzi, "How to Improve Embryos' Quality in the IVF Lab," presentation at the 24th World Congress on Controversies in Obstetrics, Gynecology & Infertility (COGI), Amsterdam, Netherlands, November 11, 2016.

8. Q. Lai, H. Zhang, G. Zhu, et al., "Comparison of the GnRH Agonist and Antagonist Protocol on the Same Patients in Assisted Reproduction During Controlled Ovarian Stimulation Cycles," *International Journal of Clinical and Experimental Pathology* 6, no. 9 (August 15, 2013):1903–10.

9. Richard Sherbahn and Michelle Catenacci, "High Live Birth Rates in IVF High Responders Using Either a Lupron Trigger Alone (Agonist Trigger) or Using a Dual Trigger if Intensive Luteal Support Is Given," research study presented by Richard Sherbahn, MD, at the 70th Annual Meeting of the American Society for Reproductive Medicine, Honolulu, October 2014.

10. A 2007 study indicated that early embryos were no better off in the uterus than in the incubator. G. Sher, L. Keskintepe, M. Keskintepe, et al., "Oocyte Karyotyping by Comparative Genomic Hybrydization Provides a

Highly Reliable Method for Selecting 'Competent' Embryos, Markedly Improving In Vitro Fertilization Outcome: A Multiphase Study," *Fertility and Sterility* 87, no. 5 (May 2007): 1033–40.

11. At one top clinic in Chicago, for example, 68.9 percent of women aged thirty-eight to forty became pregnant and 52 percent had a live birth following a blastocyst transfer, as opposed to a 40.9 percent pregnancy rate and 27.4 percent birth rate resulting from an embryo transfer. Among women just a couple of years older, aged forty-one to forty-two, the blastocyst transfers resulted in a 59.5 percent pregnancy and 37 percent live birth rate, as compared to 24.6 percent and 15.8 percent, respectively, for those who had an embryo transfer. Richard Sherbahn, "IVF Success Rates with 5 Day Blastocyst Transfers at the Advance Fertility Center of Chicago," Advanced Fertility Center of Chicago, accessed December 11, 2017, www.advancedfertility.com/blastocystpregnancyrates.htm.

12. John Rock, "Conception in a Watch Glass," *New England Journal of Medicine* 217, no. 678 (October 21, 1937).

13. A. H. Handyside, E. H. Kontogianni, K. Hardy, and R. M. Winston, "Pregnancies from Biopsied Human Preimplantation Embryos Sexed by Y-specific DNA Amplification," *Nature* 344, no. 6,268 (April 19, 1990): 768–70.

14. A. H. Handyside, J. G. Lesko, J. J. Tarin, et al., "Birth of a Normal Girl After In Vitro Fertilization and Preimplantation Diagnostic Testing for Cystic Fibrosis," *New England Journal of Medicine* 327, no. 13 (September 24, 1992): 905–9.

15. Ibid.

16. Mark Hughes, "Current and Future Molecular Diagnostic Technologies for PGS and PGD," presentation at ART World Congress, October 13, 2016.

17. Ibid.

18. L. Rienzi, A. Capalbo, M. Stoppa, et al., "No Evidence of Association Between Blastocyst Aneuploidy and Morphokinetic Assessment in a Selected Population of Poor-Prognosis Patients: A Longitudinal Cohort Study," *Reproductive BioMedicine Online* 30, no. 1 (January 2015): 57–66; R. R. Angell, A. A. Templeton, and R. J. Aitken, "Chromosome Studies in Human In Vitro Fertilization," *Human Genetics* 72, no. 4 (April 1986): 333–39.

19. See S. Mastenbroek, M. Twisk, J. van Echten-Arends, et al., "In Vitro Fertilization with Preimplantation Genetic Screening," *New England Journal of Medicine*, no. 357 (2007): 9–17.

20. Ibid.

21. Santiago Munné and Dagan Wells, "Detection of Mosaicism at Blastocyst Stage with the Use of High-Resolution Next-Generation Sequencing," *Fertility and Sterility* 107, no. 5 (May 2017): 1085–91.

22. S. Munné, "Preimplantation Genetic Diagnosis for Aneuploidy and Translocations Using Array Comparative Genomic Hybridization," *Current Genomics* 13, no. 6 (September 2012): 463–70. The first baby conceived in the UK after using aCGH was born in 2010. University of Oxford, "First IVF Babies Born Using New Chromosome Counting Technique," February 4, 2011, http://www.ox.ac.uk/news/2011-02-04-first-ivf-babies-born -using-new-chromosome-counting-technique.

23. Analysis of 15,033 embryos biopsied showed 47.3 percent to be normal (euploid), 39 percent to be abnormal (aneuploid), and 13.7 percent to be mosaic, with nearly 5 percent of the mosaics showing low levels of mosaicism and therefore treated as normal, and just under 9 percent showing high levels of abnormality. Ibid. A further analysis of data from Reprogenetics and Genesis Genetics through March 2016 regarding 33,236 embryos showed a range of mosaic embryos from 11 percent to 22 percent, depending on the age group, and a range of aneuploidy embryos from 16 percent to 42 percent. Approximately 30 percent of blastocyst-stage embryos are mosaic. Munné and Wells, "Detection of Mosaicism."

24. Hughes, "Molecular Diagnostic Technologies" presentation. Similarly, an embryo indicated as normal using aCGH was found to be a high-level mosaic, with 70 percent of its cells having trisomy 16. Santiago Munné, "An Appraisal of PGS Outcome-Data from the Two Largest PGS Providers," presentation at ART World Congress, October 13, 2016.

25. Ibid.

26. E. Greco, M. G. Minasi, and F. Florentino, "Healthy Babies After Intrauterine Transfer of Mosaic Aneuploid Blastocysts," *New England Journal of Medicine* no. 373 (2015): 2089–90.

27. Reprogenetics and Recombine, a company founded by Dr. Munné that provides carrier screening tests for couples planning to conceive, were acquired in 2015 and 2016, respectively, by CooperSurgical, and are now part of CooperGenomics, where Dr. Munné serves as chief scientific officer.

28. Stephen S. Hall, "A New Last Chance: There Could Soon Be a Baby-Boom

Among Women Who Thought They'd Hit an IVF Dead End," The Cut, *New York Magazine*, September 17, 2017, https://www.thecut.com/2017/09/ivf-abnormal-embryos-new-last-chance.html.

29. Ibid.

30. Evidence that mosaic embryos implant less than those that are euploid comes from a recent study in which mosaic embryos, as determined with the use of hrNGS, resulted in 30.1 percent initial implantations and 15.4 percent ongoing pregnancies, significantly less than a well-matched nonmosaic euploid control group (55.8 percent implantations, 46.2 percent ongoing pregnancies). Another study showed a miscarriage rate of 55.6 percent for blastocysts classified as mosaic, versus 17.2 percent for euploid control samples (Munné and Wells, "Detection of Mosaicism").

31. Ibid.

32. Pasquale Patrizio, head of fertility medicine at Yale University, and Sherman Silber of St. Luke's Hospital in St. Louis, quoted in Hall, "New Last Chance."

33. Z. Yang, J. Liu, G. S. Collins, et al., "Selection of Single Blastocysts for Fresh Transfer Via Standard Morphology Assessment Alone and with Array CGH for Good Prognosis IVF Patients: Results from a Randomized Pilot Study," *Molecular Cytogenetics* 5, no. 1 (May 2, 2012): 24; R. T. Scott, K. M. Upham, E. J. Forman, et al., "Blastocyst Biopsy with Comprehensive Chromosome Screening and Fresh Embryo Transfer Significantly Increases In Vitro Fertilization Implantation and Delivery Rates: A Randomized Controlled Trial," *Fertility and Sterility* 100, no. 3 (September 2013): 697–703; E. J. Forman et al., "In Vitro Fertilization with Single Euploid Blastocyst Transfer: A Randomized Controlled Trial," *Fertility and Sterility* 100, no. 1 (July 2013): 100–7.

34. E. M. Dahdouh, J. Balayla, and J. A. Garcia-Velasco, "Impact of Blastocyst Biopsy and Comprehensive Chromosome Screening Technology on Preimplantation Genetic Screening: A Systematic Review of Randomized Controlled Trials," *Reproductive BioMedicine Online* 30, no. 3 (March 2015): 281–89; E. Lee, P. Illingworth, L. Wilton, and G. M. Chambers, "The Clinical Effectiveness of Preimplantation Genetic Diagnosis for Aneuploidy in All 24 Chromosomes (PGD-A): Systematic Review," *Human Reproduction* 30, no. 2 (February 2015): 473–83.

35. J. Chang, S. L. Boulet, G. Jeng, et al., "Outcomes of In Vitro Fertilization

with Preimplantation Genetic Diagnosis: An Analysis of the United States Assisted Reproductive Technology Surveillance Data, 2011–2012," *Fertility and Sterility* 105, no. 2 (February 2016): 394–400.

36. G. Murugappan, L. Shahine, C. Perfetto, et al., "Intent to Treat Analysis of *In Vitro* Fertilization and Preimplantation Genetic Screening Versus Expectant Management in Patients with Recurrent Pregnancy Loss," *Human Reproduction* 31, no. 8 (August 1, 2016): 1668–74.

37. SART 2014 National Summary Report, https://www.sartcorsonline.com/rptCSR_PublicMultYear.aspx.

38. G. L. Harton, S. Munné, M. Surrey, et al., "Diminished Effect of Maternal Age on Implantation after Preimplantation Genetic Diagnosis with Array Comparative Genomic Hybridization," *Fertility and Sterility* 100, no. 6 (December 2013):1695–703.

39. SART 2014; Munné "Appraisal of PGS Outcome-Data" presentation.

40. Jacques Cohen, "Design and quality control of future IVF laboratories," presentation at 2016 ART World Congress, October 14, 2016.

Chapter 8

1. Kate Wighton, "Miscarriage and Ectopic Pregnancy May Trigger Post-Traumatic Stress Disorder," Imperial College London, November 2, 1016, http://www3.imperial.ac.uk/newsandeventspggrp/imperialcollege/newssummary/news_1-11-2016-17-15-45.

2. March of Dimes, "Miscarriage," http://www.marchofdimes.org/complications/miscarriage.aspx.

3. For an exceptional examination of miscarriage, see Jon Cohen, *Coming to Term: Uncovering the Truth About Miscarriage* (New Brunswick, NJ: Rutgers University Press, 2007). The statistics cited herein can be found on page 16.

4. Mark Hughes, "Molecular Diagnostic Technologies" presentation.

5. Together with Lord Robert Winston and Dr. Alan Handyside.

6. Murugappan et al., "Intent to Treat Analysis."

7. See chapter 13, particularly "Improving Egg Quality through Hormones: The Pregmama Story," for an in-depth discussion of research into improving egg quality.

8. Diethylstilbestrol, a synthetic estrogen known as DES, became a popular treatment for the prevention of miscarriage from the late 1940s to the

early 1970s, despite a lack of controlled studies demonstrating its efficacy or serious investigation of its safety for mother or child. Amid mounting concern about both, in 1971, the FDA advised doctors to stop prescribing DES to pregnant women. Beginning in the 1970s, significant research emerged revealing a troubling number of serious problems: DES caused clear cell adenocarcinoma in some women who took it; uterine abnormalities in as many as a third of the daughters born to mothers who took it, which led to devastatingly high miscarriage and infertility rates; an increased risk of breast cancer among mothers who took it; and rubbing salt in the wound, actually increased the risk of miscarriage in mothers who took it. For a thorough examination of the history and effects of DES, see Jon Cohen, *Coming to Term*, 116–29.

9. While a certain genetic problem called a "balanced translocation" in either parent is also known to cause recurrent miscarriage, there is unfortunately no treatment for this condition, and intended parents who are diagnosed with this are advised to seek genetic counseling.

10. Jon Cohen, *Coming to Term*, 113.

11. R. Rai, M. Backos, F. Rushworth, and L. Regan, "Polycystic Ovaries and Recurrent Miscarriage—A Reappraisal," *Human Reproduction* 15, no. 3 (March 1, 2000): 612–15.

12. J. X. Wang, M. J. Davies, and R. J. Norman, "Polycystic Ovarian Syndrome and the Risk of Spontaneous Abortion Following Assisted Reproduction Technology Treatment," *Human Reproduction* 16 (2001): 2606–9.

13. R. S. Legro, H. X. Barnhart, W. D. Schlaff, et al., "Clomiphene, Metformin, or Both for Infertility in the Polycystic Ovary Syndrome," *New England Journal of Medicine*, February 356, no. 6 (2007): 551–66.

14. E. Moll, P. M. Bossuyt, J. C. Korevaar, et al., "Effect of Clomifene Citrate Plus Metformin and Clomifene Citrate Plus Placebo on Induction of Ovulation in Women with Newly Diagnosed Polycystic Ovary Syndrome: Randomised Double Blind Clinical Trial," *BMJ* 332, no. 7,556 (Jun 24):1485.

15. E. Vanky, S. Stridsklev, R. Heimstad, et al., "Metformin versus Placebo from First Trimester to Delivery in Polycystic Ovary Syndrome: A Randomized, Controlled Multicenter Study," *Journal of Clinical Endocrinology & Metabolism* 95, no. 12 (December 2010): e448–55.

16. V. De Leo, M. C. Musacchio, P. Piomboni, et al., "The Administration of Metformin During Pregnancy Reduces Polycystic Ovary Syndrome

Related Gestational Complications," *European Journal of Obstetrics and Gynecology and Reproductive Biology* 157, no. 1 (July 2011): 63–66. See also F. H. Nawaz, R. Khalid, T. Naru, and J. Rizvi, "Does Continuous Use of Metformin throughout Pregnancy Improve Pregnancy Outcomes in Women with Polycystic Ovarian Syndrome?," *Journal of Obstetrics and Gynaecology Research* 34, no. 5 (October 2008): 832–37.

17. T. B. Mesen and S. L. Young, "Progesterone and the Luteal Phase: A Requisite to Reproduction," *Obstetrics and Gynecology Clinics of North America* 42, no. 1 (March 2015): 135–51; P. Miller and M. Soules, "Luteal Phase Deficiency: Pathophysiology, Diagnosis and Treatment," *Global Library of Women's Medicine*, May 2009.

18. Jon Cohen, *Coming to Term*, 108.

19. R. M. Oates-Whitehead, D. Haas, and J. Carrier, "Progesterone for Preventing Miscarriage," *Cochrane Database of Systematic Reviews*, no. 4 (October 20, 2003): article ID CD003511. Updated by D. M. Haas and P. S. Ramsey, "Progesterone for Preventing Miscarriage," *Cochrane Database of Systematic Reviews*, no. 2 (April 16, 2008): article ID CD003511, and D. M. Haas and P. S. Ramsey, "Progesterone for Preventing Miscarriage," *Cochrane Database of Systematic Reviews*, no. 10 (October 31, 2013): article ID CD003511.

20. A. Coomarasamy, H. Williams, E. Truchanowicz, et al., "PROMISE: First-Trimester Progesterone Therapy in Women with a History of Unexplained Recurrent Miscarriages—a Randomised, Double-Blind, Placebo-Controlled, International Multicentre Trial and Economic Evaluation," *Health Technology Assessment* 20, no. 41 (May 2016): 1–92.

21. Mayo Clinic, "Cervical Cerclage," March 17, 2015, http://www.mayo clinic.org/tests-procedures/cervical-cerclage/basics/definition/prc -20012949.

22. S. M. Althuisius, G. A. Dekker, P. Hummel, and H. P. van Gejin, "Cervical Incompetence Prevention Randomized Cerclage Trial: Emergency Cerclage with Bed Rest versus Bed Rest Alone," *American Journal of Obstetrics & Gynecology* 189, no. 4 (October 2003): 907–10.

23. See A. O. Rust, R. O. Atlas, K. J. Jones, et al., "A Randomized Trial of Cerclage versus No Cerclage among Patients with Ultasonographically Detected Second-Trimester Peterm Dilation of the Internal Os," *American Journal of Obstetrics & Gynecology* 183 (October 2000): 830–85; A. J. Drakeley, D. Roberts, and Z. Alfirevic, "Cervical Cerclage for Prevention

of Preterm Delivery: Meta-analysis of Randomized Trials," *Obstetrics & Gynecology* 102, no. 3 (September 2003): 621–27.

24. V. Berghella, T. J. Rafael, J. M. Szychowski, et al., "Cerclage for Short Cervix on Ultrasonography in Women with Singleton Gestations and Previous Preterm Birth: A Meta-analysis," *Obstetrics & Gynecology* 117, no. 3 (March 2011): 663–71.

25. T. J. Rafael, V. Berghella, and Z. Alfirevic, "Cervical Stitch (Cerclage) for Preventing Preterm Birth in Multiple Pregnancy," *Cochrane Database of Systematic Reviews*, no. 9 (September 2014): article ID CD009166.

26. APS Support UK, "About APS—Pregancy," accessed December 11, 2017, http://www.aps-support.org.uk/about-aps/pregnancy.php.

27. R. S. Rai, L. Regan, K. Clifford, et al., "Immunology: Antiphospholipid Antibodies and β2-Glycoprotein-I in 500 Women with Recurrent Miscarriage: Results of a Comprehensive Screening Approach, *Human Reproduction* 10, no. 8 (August 1, 1995): 2001–5.

28. R. Rai, H. Cohen, M. Dave, and L. Regan, "Randomised Controlled Trial of Aspirin and Aspirin Plus Heparin in Pregnant Women with Recurrent Miscarriage Associated with Phospholipid Antibodies (or Antiphospholipid Antibodies)," *BMJ* 314, no 7,706 (January 25, 1997):253–57.

29. Megan Brooks, "Pravastatin Shows Promise in Pregnant Women with Antiphospholipid Syndrome," Reuters Health, August 1, 2016, https://www.consultant360.com/story/pravastatin-shows-promise-pregnant-women-antiphospholipid-syndrome.

30. Reproductive Immunology Associates, "Miscarriages Can Be Prevented," accessed December 11, 2017, http://www.rialab.com/fertility-services/reproductive-immunology/multiple-miscarriages-can-be-prevented.php; Braverman IVF & Reproductive Immunology, "Patients with 5 or more miscarriages have an outstanding 80% chance of having a successful pregnancy with our treatment protocols (all pregnancies delivered or currently past 20 weeks). A review of 30 cases at Braverman IVF & Reproductive Immunology," posted on June 23, 2015, http://www.preventmiscarriage.com/patients-with-5-or-more-miscarriages-have-an-out.html.

31. Jon Cohen, *Coming to Term*, 64–66.

32. Peter Castro and Giovanna Breu, "Injection of Hope," *People*, October 28, 1996, http://people.com/archive/injection-of-hope-vol-46-no-18/.

33. Jerry Adler, Susan Katz, Elisa Williams, and Vicki Quade, "Learning from the Loss," *Newsweek*, March 24, 1986, 66.

34. B. Stray-Pedersen and S. Stray-Pedersen, "Etiologic Factors and Subsequent Reproductive Performance in 195 Couples with a Prior History of Habitual Abortion," *American Journal of Obstetrics & Gynecology* 148, no. 2 (January 15, 1984):140–46. See also Jon Cohen, *Coming to Term*, 175–77.

35. H. S. Liddell, N. S. Pattison, and A. Zanderigo, "Recurrent Miscarriage—Outcome After Supportive Care in Early Pregnancy," *Australian and New Zealand Journal of Obstetrics and Gynaecology* 31, no. 4 (November 1991): 320–22.

36. C. Ober, T. Karrison, R. Odem, et al., "Mononuclear-cell immunisation in prevention of recurrent miscarriages: a randomised trial," *The Lancet* 354, no. 9176 (July 31, 1999): 365–69.

37. Department of Health and Human Services, Public Health Service, Food and Drug Administration, "Lymphocyte Immune Therapy (LIT) Letter," January 30, 2002, https://wayback.archive-it.org/7993/20170406072912/https://www.fda.gov/BiologicsBloodVaccines/SafetyAvailability/ucm105848.htm.

38. A. Moffett, L. Regan, and P. Braude, "Natural Killer Cells, Miscarriage, and Infertility," *BMJ* 329, no. 7,477 (November 27, 2004): 1283–85.

39. L. F. Wong, T. Porter, and J. R. Scott, "Immunotherapy for Recurrent Miscarriage," *Cochrane Database of Systematic Reviews*, no. 10 (2014): article ID CD000112.

40. Geoffrey Sher, "IVIG & Intralipid Therapy in IVF: Interpreting Natural Killer Cell Activity for Diagnosis and Treatment," *Doctors Blog*, Sher Fertility, https://haveababy.com/fertility-information/ivf-authority/ivig-intralipid-therapy-in-ivf-natural-killer-cell-activity-for-diagnosis-and-treatment. In the interest of full disclosure, my daughter, Alexandra, was conceived under the care of Dr. Batzofin at Sher Fertility, although without immunology treatment.

41. Braverman IVF & Reproductive Immunology, "IVIG Treatment for Miscarriages" accessed December 11, 2017, http://www.preventmiscarriage.com/intravenous-immunoglobulin-ivig-.html.

42. Alan E. Beer, Julia Kantecki, and Jane Reed, *Is Your Body Baby Friendly?: "Unexplained" Infertility, Miscarriage & IVF Failure* (Leesburg, VA: AJR Publishing, 2006), 4.

43. A. J. Wilcox, C. R. Weinberg, J. F. O'Connor, et al., "Incidence of Early
Loss of Pregnancy," *New England Journal of Medicine* 319, no. 4 (July 28,
1988) 189–94; R. M. Lee and R. M. Silver, "Recurrent Pregnancy Loss:
Summary and Clinical Recommendations," *Seminars in Reproductive Medicine* 18, no. 4 (2000): 433–40. See also "Getting Pregnant—Pregnancy
After Miscarriage: What You Need to Know," Mayo Clinic, http://www
.mayoclinic.org/healthy-lifestyle/getting-pregnant/in-depth/pregnancy
-after-miscarriage/art-20044134; "After a Miscarriage: Getting Pregnant Again," American Pregnancy Association, http://americanpregnancy
.org/pregnancy-loss/after-miscarriage-getting-pregnant-again/.

Chapter 9

1. E. Scott Sills, ed., *Handbook of Gestational Surrogacy: International Clinical
Practice and Policy Issues* (Cambridge, UK: Cambridge University Press,
2016), 1.
2. W. H. Utian, L. A. Sheean, J. M. Goldfarb, and R. Kiwi, "Successful Pregnancy After In Vitro Fertilization and Embryo Transfer from an Infertile
Woman to a Surrogate," *New England Journal of Medicine* 313, no. 21 (November 21, 1985):1351–52.
3. For a detailed exploration of laws in different countries, see Sills, *Handbook*.
4. The Surrogacy Experience, "U.S. Surrogacy Laws by State," http://www
.thesurrogacyexperience.com/u-s-surrogacy-law-by-state.html.
5. Alexandra Sifferlin, "Battle Over Paid Surrogacy Opens New Front," *Time*,
January 28, 2015, http://time.com/3666606/battle-over-paid-surrogacy
-opens-new-front/; Anemona Hartocollis, "And Surrogacy Makes 3: In
New York, a Push for Compensated Surrogacy," *New York Times*, February 19, 2014, https://www.nytimes.com/2014/02/20/fashion/In-New
-York-Some-Couples-Push-for-Legalization-of-Compensated-Surrogacy
.html?_r=0.
6. Quoted in A. S. Persky, "Reproductive Technology and the Law," *Washington Lawyer*, July/August 2012, https://www.dcbar.org/bar-resources
/publications/washington-lawyer/articles/july-august-2012-reproduc
tive-tech.cfm.
7. Ibid.

Chapter 10

1. Jacqueline Mroz, "One Sperm Donor, 150 Offspring," *New York Times*, September 5, 2011, http://www.nytimes.com/2011/09/06/health/06donor.html?_r=0. For an excellent discussion of this and other aspects of sperm donation, see Jacqueline Mroz, *Scattered Seeds: In Search of Family and Identity in the Sperm Donor Generation* (Berkeley, CA: Seal Press, 2017).

2. Mroz, "One Sperm Donor."

3. Mroz, *Scattered Seeds*, 177.

4. A. Tanaka, M. Nagayoshi, I, Tanaka, et al., "Controversy Over Rights of Children Born from Oocyte Donations, Is Full Disclosure of Donor's Identity Necessary?," *Fertility and Sterility* 104, no. 3 (September 2015): e231

5. Kristen Riggan, "Regulation (or Lack Thereof) of Assisted Reproductive Technologies in the U.S. and Abroad," Center for Bioethics & Human Dignity, March 4, 2011, https://cbhd.org/content/regulation-or-lack-thereof-assisted-reproductive-technologies-us-and-abroad. See also Mroz, *Scattered Seeds*, 164.

6. D. A. Greenfeld and S. C. Klock, "Disclosure Decisions among Known and Anonymous Oocyte Donation Recipients," *Fertility and Sterility* 81, no. 6 (June 2004): 1565–71.

7. Dr. Joan Manheimer, interview with the author, April 1, 2016.

8. Nancy Hass, "To Tell, or Not to Tell, Your Egg Donor Baby?" *Elle*, August 20, 2015, http://www.elle.com/life-love/sex-relationships/news/a29904/whose-life-is-it-anyway/.

9. Quoted in Hass, "To Tell."

10. Wendy Kramer, "The Ethical Sperm Bank: An All-Open Sperm Bank. An Idea Whose Time Has Come," The Blog, *Huffington Post*, July 22, 2015, updated July 22, 2016, https://www.huffingtonpost.com/wendy-kramer/the-ethical-sperm-bank-an_b_7841180.html.

11. Donor Sibling Registry statistics, as of October 13, 2017, found at https://donorsiblingregistry.com.

12. Mroz, "One Sperm Donor." See also Mroz, *Scattered Seeds*, chapter 8.

13. Wendy Kramer, "A Brief History of Donor Conception," *The Huffington Post*, May 10, 2016, https://www.huffingtonpost.com/wendy-kramer/a-brief

-history-of-donor-conception_b_9814184.html; Mroz, *Scattered Seeds*, 79–85.

14. Mroz, *Scattered Seeds*, 77–78, 89–103.

15. At the Sperm Bank of California, which tracks its donor-conceived births, 60 percent of the children are born to lesbian parents and 20 percent to single mothers. Mroz, *Scattered Seeds*, 109.

16. Tamar Lewin, "Sperm Banks Accused of Losing Samples and Lying About Donors," *New York Times*, July 21, 2016, https://www.nytimes.com /2016/07/22/us/sperm-banks-accused-of-losing-samples-and-lying -about-donors.html?_r=0.

17. Ibid.

18. Ibid.

19. Theresa Boyle, "U.S. Sperm Bank Admits It Doesn't Verify Donor Information," *The Star*, April 9, 2015, https://www.thestar.com/life /health_wellness/2015/04/09/us-sperm-bank-sued-by-canadian-couple -says-it-didnt-verify-donor-information.html.

20. Mroz, *Scattered Seeds*, 176–77.

21. "Success Stories," Donor Sibling Registry, https://donorsiblingregistry .com/success-stories.

22. Mroz, *Scattered Seeds*, 56–63.

23. Hass, "To Tell."

Chapter 11

1. Arkansas, California, Connecticut, Hawaii, Illinois, Louisiana, Maryland, Massachusetts, Montana, New Jersey, New York, Ohio, Rhode Island, Texas, and West Virginia. See "Coverage by State," Resolve: The National Infertility Association, accessed December 11, 2017, http://resolve.org /what-are-my-options/insurance-coverage/coverage-state/.

2. Arkansas, Hawaii, Maryland, and Texas. Ibid.

3. The Fertility Clinic Success Rate and Certification Act of 1992 (FCSRCA, or Public Law 102-493) requires that clinics performing ART annually provide data for all procedures performed to the CDC. The CDC is required to use these data to report and publish clinic-specific success rates and certification of embryo laboratories.

4. US Department of Health and Human Services Centers for Disease

Control and Prevention, *2006 Assisted Reproductive Technology Success Rates: National Summary and Fertility Clinic Reports* (Atlanta: CDC, 2008).

5. See Riggan, "Regulation (or Lack Thereof)."
6. PBS *Frontline* interview with Dr. Mark Sauer, accessed December 11, 2017, http://www.pbs.org/wgbh/pages/frontline/shows/fertility/interviews/sauer.html.
7. See J. Johnston, M. K. Gusmano, and P. Patrizio, "Preterm Births, Multiples, and Fertility Treatment: Recommendations for Changes to Policy and Clinical Practices," *Fertility and Sterility* 102, no. 1 (July 2014): 36–39.
8. Ibid, 36.
9. Ibid, 38.
10. Sumathi Reddy, "Fertility Study Warns of Risks from Multiple Births," *Wall Street Journal*, April 28, 2014, https://www.wsj.com/articles/fertility-study-warns-of-risks-from-1398726124; Bernice Yeung and Jonathan Jones, "When Pregnancy Dreams Become IVF Nightmares," Reveal: from the Center for Investigative Reporting, https://www.revealnews.org/article/when-pregnancy-dreams-become-ivf-nightmares/.
11. Quoted in Yeung and Jones, "Pregnancy Dreams."
12. The Ethics Committee of the American Society for Reproductive Medicine, "Financial Compensation of Oocyte Donors," *Fertility and Sterility* 88, no. 1 (August 2007): 305.
13. US Department of Health and Human Services Centers for Disease Control and Prevention, *2013 Assisted Reproductive Technology National Summary Report* (Atlanta: CDC, 2015).
14. Defendants' Motion to Dismiss Plaintiff's First Amended Class Action Complaint, Kamakahi v. Am. Soc'y for Reprod. Med., 305 F.R.D. 164 (N.D. Cal. 2015) (No. 11–cv–01781–JCS), 2011.
15. Quoted in Lewin, "Sperm Banks Accused."
16. Tamar Lewin, "Egg Donors Challenge Pay Rates, Saying They Shortchange Women," *New York Times*, October 16, 2015, https://www.nytimes.com/2015/10/17/us/egg-donors-challenge-pay-rates-saying-they-shortchange-women.html.
17. Lindsay Kamakahi, Justine Levy, Chelsea Kimmel, and Kristin Wells.
18. Class Action Complaint, Kamakahi v. Am. Soc'y for Reprod. Med., 305 F.R.D. 164 (N.D. Cal. 2015) (No. 11–cv–01781–JCS), 2011.
19. The settlement also provides for payment to plaintiffs' lawyers in the

amount of $1.5 million, and compensation to each of the four named plaintiffs in the amount of $5,000. See Jacob Gershman, "Fertility Industry Group Settles Lawsuit Over Egg Donor Price Caps," *Wall Street Journal*, February 3, 2016, https://blogs.wsj.com/law/2016/02/03/fertility-industry-group-settles-lawsuit-over-egg-donor-price-caps/; Melissa LaFreniere, "Egg Donors Get Price Cap Removed in Class Action Lawsuit Settlement," *Top Class Actions*, February 2, 2016, https://topclassactions.com/lawsuit-settlements/lawsuit-news/327105-egg-donors-get-price-cap-removed-in-class-action-lawsuit-settlement/. The current ASRM guidelines can be found at http://www.asrm.org/globalassets/asrm/asrm-content/news-and-publications/ethics-committee-opinions/financial_compensation_of_oocyte_donors-pdfmembers.pdf.

20. Quoted in Lewin, "Egg Donors Challenge."

21. R. H. Reindollar, M. M. Regan, P. J. Neumann, et al., "A Randomized Clinical Trial to Evaluate Optimal Treatment for Unexplained Infertility: The Fast Track and Standard Treatment (FASTT) Trial," *Fertility and Sterility* 94, no. 3 (August 2010): 888–99.

22. American Cancer Society, "What Are the Risk Factors for Ovarian Cancer?," accessed December 17, 2017, https://www.cancer.org/cancer/ovarian-cancer/causes-risks-prevention/risk-factors.html; F. Tomao, G. Lo Russo, G. P. Spinelli, et al., "Fertility Drugs, Reproductive Strategies and Ovarian Cancer Risk," *Journal of Ovarian Research,* no. 7 (2014): 51.

23. Quoted in Michael Ollove, "Lightly Regulated In Vitro Fertilization Yields Thousands of Babies Annually," *Washington Post*, April 13, 2015, https://www.washingtonpost.com/national/health-science/lightly-regulated-in-vitro-fertilization-yields-thousands-of-babies-annually/2015/04/13/f1f3fa36-d8a2-11e4-8103-fa84725dbf9d_story.html?utm_term=.026bd065d982. Debra Mathews of the Johns Hopkins Berman Institute of Bioethics agrees that "assisted reproduction has grown up as a medical services business, not under the auspices of medical research."

24. For a discussion of early attempts to cure infertility, see Spar, *Baby Business*, 17–24.

25. Paul Ramsey, *Fabricated Man: The Ethics of Genetic Control* (New Haven, CT: Yale University Press, 1970), 138.

26. Quoted in Ollove, "Lightly Regulated."

27. "Obama Overturns Bush Policy on Stem Cell," CNN News, March 9,

2009, http://www.cnn.com/2009/POLITICS/03/09/obama.stem
.cells/; H. Wolinsky, "The Pendulum Swung. President Barack Obama
Removes Restrictions on Stem-Cell Research, but Are Expectations Now
Too High?" *EMBO Reports* 10, no. 5 (May 2009): 436–39.

28. Megan Kearl, "Dickey-Wicker Amendment, 1996," *The Embryo Project Ency-
clopedia*, https://embryo.asu.edu/pages/dickey-wicker-amendment-1996.

29. E. R. Myers, D. C. McCrory, A. A. Mills, et al., "Effectiveness of Assisted
Reproductive Technology (ART)," *Evidence Report/Technology Assessment*,
no. 167 (May 2008):1–195.

30. See chapter 14, notes 17–19.

Chapter 12

1. Marketdata Enterprises, "U.S. Fertility Clinics & Infertility Services:
An Industry Analysis," October 2013, https://www.marketdataenter
prises.com/wp-content/uploads/2014/01/Infertility%20Services%20
Mkt%202013%20TOC.pdf.

2. See Rene Letourneau, "Global Infertility Drugs, Devices Market to
Approach $4.8B in 2017," *Healthcare Finance*, October 3, 2012; Cat
Zakrzewski, "VCs See Opportunity in Growing Fertility Market," *Wall
Street Journal*, February 7, 2017, https://www.wsj.com/articles/vcs-see
-opportunity-in-growing-fertility-market-1486470601.

3. According to the ASRM. See http://www.reproductivefacts.org/faqs
/frequently-asked-questions-about-infertility/q06-is-in-vitro-fertiliza
tion-expensive/.

4. According to FertilityIQ. See https://www.fertilityiq.com/cost.

5. Ibid.

6. Ibid.

7. P. Katz, J. Showstack, J. Smith, et al., "Costs of Infertility Treatment: Results from an 18-Month Prospective Cohort Study," *Fertility and Sterility*
95, no. 3 (March 1, 2011): 915–21.

8. See chapter 11, note 1.

9. Katz et al., "Costs of Infertility Treatment."

10. Fertility lenders such as CapexMD offer loans through participating fertility clinics.

11. See FertilityIQ, "Paying for IVF with a Loan or Credit Card," accessed

December 11, 2017, https://www.fertilityiq.com/cost/paying-for-ivf -with-a-loan-or-credit-card.

12. Attain IVF, "Multi-Cycle Programs Overview," accessed December 11, 2017, http://attainivf.attainfertility.com/attain-ivf-flex-plan-overview. Attain IVF offers its Muti-Cycle Programs exclusively through clinics and physicians within the nationwide network of IntegraMed Fertility.

13. ARC Fertility, "The ARC Success Program," accessed December 11, 2017, https://www.arcfertility.com/arc-treatment-packages/the-arc-success -program/. ARC Fertility operates through a nationwide network of doctors and clinics, offering referrals, treatment packages—such as the ARC Success Program and ARC Cycle Plus Programs—and financing options, through ARC Fertility Financing.

14. See FertilityIQ, "IVF Refund and Package Programs," accessed December 11, 2017, https://www.fertilityiq.com/cost/ivf-refund-and-pack age-programs.

15. Ibid.

16. Dean Kirby, "Couples to Get 'Money Back Guarantee' on IVF treatment," *Manchester Evening News* (UK), July 31, 2014, http://www.manches tereveningnews.co.uk/news/greater-manchester-news/money-back -failed-ivf-fertility-7545779.

17. See Access Fertility homepage, www.accessfertility.co.uk.

18. Ginia Bellafonte, "Baby-Making by Lottery," *New York Times*, April 27, 2017, https://www.nytimes.com/2017/04/27/nyregion/zhang-fertil ity-center-lottery.html.

19. *Frontline* interview with Sauer.

20. Quoted in "The Fertility Race: The Fertility Industry—Business Is Prospering," American RadioWorks, American Public Media, accessed December 11, 2017, http://americanradioworks.publicradio.org/features /fertility_race/part3/section1.shtml.

21. Quoted in Spar, *Baby Business*, 46.

22. Ibid, 50.

23. See Fred Decker, "The Salaries of Fertility Doctors," *Houston Chronicle*, accessed December 11, 2017, http://work.chron.com/salaries-fertility -doctors-3463.html.

24. *Frontline* interview with Sauer.

25. Fertility Authority, "IVF Success Rates May Be Misleading," accessed De-

cember 11, 2017, https://www.fertilityauthority.com/articles/ivf-suc
cess-rates-may-be-misleading; V. A. Kushnir, A. Vidali, D. H. Barad, and
N. Gleicher, "The Status of Public Reporting of Clinical Outcomes in Assisted Reproductive Technology," *Fertility and Sterility* 100, no. 3 (September 2013): 736–41.

26. CDC, *2013 Assisted Reproductive Technology*, 5.

27. "IVF Success Rates May be Misleading."

28. Press Association, "Fertility Treatments 'Threaten Our Humanity,' Warns
Robert Winston," *The Guardian*, May 5, 2014, https://www.theguard
ian.com/science/2014/may/05/fertility-treatments-threaten-humanity
-winston. Lord Winston was formerly president of the British Association
for the Advancement of Science.

29. F. Bissonette, S. J. Phillips, J. Gunby, et al., "Working to Eliminate Multiple
Pregnancies: A Success Story in Québec," *Reproductive BioMedicine Online*
23, no. 4 (October 2011): 500–4.

30. This view is supported by a paper that came out of a March of Dimes–
supported research project that involved a comprehensive review of medical, policy, and ethics literature and a workshop with leading clinicians,
professional association leaders, patient advocates, and insurance industry
representatives. See Johnston et al., "Preterm Births."

31. Survey by Mercer Health and Benefits LLC, "Employer Experience with,
and Attitudes Toward, Coverage of Infertility Treatment," May 31, 2006,
http://familybuilding.resolve.org/site/DocServer/Mercer_-_Resolve
_Final_report.pdf?docID=4361.

32. See Johnston et al., "Preterm Births," 37.

33. E. G. Hughes and D. Dejean "Cross-border Fertility Services in North
America: A Survey of Canadian and American Providers," *Fertility and Sterility* 94, no. 1 (June 2010): e16–19.

34. See Maria Finoshina, "Fertility Tourists Eye Russia," *RT News*, December
13, 2010, https://www.rt.com/news/fertility-tourists-eye-russia/; Tom
Parfitt, "Why Infertility Treatment Is Booming in Ukraine," *The Guardian*,
May 22, 2009, https://www.theguardian.com/world/2009/may/22
/infertility-treatment-ukraine; www.fertilityclinicsabroad.com; www
.fertility.treatmentabroad.com.

35. Business Wire, "Russia In Vitro Fertilization—Opportunity Analysis and
Industry Forecast, 2014–2022—Research and Markets," August 24, 2017,

http://www.businesswire.com/news/home/20170824005481/en
/Russia-Vitro-Fertilization—-Opportunity-Analysis-Industry.

36. At the Fertility Institutes, a group of clinics in Los Angeles, New York, and
    Mexico, nearly 90 percent of their patients come for family balancing. Su-
    mathi Reddy, "Fertility Clinics Let You Select Your Baby's Sex," *Wall Street
    Journal*, Aug 17, 2015, https://www.wsj.com/articles/fertility-clinics
    -let-you-select-your-babys-sex-1439833091.

37. For further background on Enid's story, see Persky, "Reproductive Tech-
    nology," 1–2.

Chapter 13

1. Analysis of 15,033 embryos biopsied showed 47.3 percent to be normal
   (euploid), 39 percent to be abnormal (aneuploid), and 13.7 percent to be
   mosaic, with nearly 5 percent of the mosaics showing low levels of mosaicism and therefore treated as normal, and just under 9 percent showing
   high levels of abnormality (Reddy, "Fertility Clinics"). A further analysis
   of data from Reprogenetics and Genesis Genetics through March 2016
   regarding 33,236 embryos showed a range of mosaic embryos from 11
   percent to 22 percent depending on age group, and a range of aneuploidy
   embryos from 16 percent to 42 percent.

2. Munné, "Appraisal of PGS Outcome-Data" presentation.

3. Ibid.

4. Santiago Munné, "Aneuploidy in Embryos: Variability Between Centers,
   Between Patients, and Between Cycles of the Same Patients," presentation
   at CoGen First World Congress on Controversies in Preconception, Preimplantation, and Prenatal Genetic Diagnosis: How Will Genetics Drive
   the Future?," September 25–27, 2015, http://www.ivf-worldwide.com
   /cogen/oep/pgd-pgs/aneuploidy-in-embryos-variability-between-cen
   ters,-between-patients-and-between-cycles-of-the-same-patients.html.

5. S. I. Nagaoka, T. J. Hassold, and P. A. Hunt, "Human Aneuploidy: Mechanisms and New Insights into an Age-Old Problem," *Nature Reviews Genetics*
   13, no. 7 (June 18, 2012): 493–504; E. Fragouli, S. Alfarawati, N. N. Good-
   all, et al., "The Cytogenetics of Polar Bodies: Insights into Female Meiosis
   and the Diagnosis of Aneuploidy," *Molecular Human Reproduction* 17, no. 5
   (May 2011): 286–95.

6. A. H. Handyside, M. Montag, M. C. Magli, et al., "Multiple Meiotic Errors Caused by Predivision of Chromatids in Women of Advanced Maternal Age Undergoing *In Vitro* Fertilisation," *European Journal of Human Genetics* 20, no. 7 (July 2012): 742–47; A. S. Gabriel, et al., "Array Comparative Genomic Hybridisation on First Polar Bodies Suggests That Non-disjunction Is Not the Predominant Mechanism Leading to Aneuploidy in Humans," *Journal of Medical Genetics* 48, no. 7 (July 2011): 433–37; R. R. Angell, "Predivision in Human Oocytes at Meiosis I: A Mechanism for Trisomy Formation in Man," *Human Genetics* 86, no. 4 (February 1991):383–87; J. M. Fisher, J. F. Harvey, N. E. Morton, and P. A. Jacobs, "Trisomy 18: Studies of the Parent and Cell Division of Origin and the Effect of Aberrant Recombination on Nondisjunction," *American Journal of Human Genetics* 56, no. 3 (March 1995): 669–75; M. Bugge, A. Collins, M. Petersen, et al., "Non-Disjunction of Chromosome 18," *Human Molecular Genetics* 7, no. 4 (April 1, 1998): 661–69; A. Kuliev and Y. Verlinsky, "Meiotic and Mitotic Nondisjunction: Lessons from Preimplantation Genetic Diagnosis," *Human Reproduction Update* 10, no. 5 (September-October 2004): 401–7.

7. Nagaoka et al., "Human Aneuploidy." Errors can also occur during subsequent stages of mitosis, when a single cell divides into two identical daughter cells.

8. P. A. Hunt and T. J. Hassold, "Human Female Meiosis: What Makes a Good Egg Go Bad?," *Trends in Genetics* 24, no. 2 (February 2008): 86–93.

9. R. M. Winston and K. Hardy, "Are We Ignoring Potential Dangers of *In Vitro* Fertilization and Related Treatments?" *Nature Cell Biology* 4, supplement (October 2002): S14–18 and *Nature Medicine* 8, supplement (October 2002): S14–18.

10. Ibid.

11. E. B. Baart, E. Martini, M. J. Eijkemans, et al., "Milder Ovarian Stimulation for In-vitro Fertilization Reduces Aneuploidy in the Human Preimplantation Embryo: A Randomized Controlled Trial," *Human Reproduction* 22, no. 4 (April 2007): 980–88.

12. C. Rubio, A. Mercader, P. Alamá, et al., "Prospective Cohort Study in High Responder Oocyte Donors Using Two Hormonal Stimulation Protocols: Impact on Embryo Aneuploidy and Development," *Human Reproduction* 25, no. 9 (September 2010): 2290–97.

13. F. Ubaldi, L. Rienzi, E. Baroni, S. Ferrero, et al., "Hopes and Facts About

Mild Ovarian Stimulation," *Reproductive BioMedicine Online* 14, no. 6 (June 2007): 675–81.

14. G. N. Allahbadia, "Stimulation and Aneuploidy: Why Are Milder Stimulation Protocols Better?," *IVF Lite* 3, no. 2 (October 14, 2016): 41–5.

15. Keiichi Kato, "Natural-Cycle IVF: 10-Year Experience," presentation at 2016 ART World Congress, October 13, 2016.

16. V. V. Grabar and A. V. Stefanovich, "Aneuploidies in Oocytes Used in IVF Programs," *Georgian Medical News*, no. 237 (December 2014): 7–12.

17. Cited in Nicholas Kristof, "Contaminating Our Bodies with Everyday Products," *New York Times*, November 28, 2015, https://www.nytimes.com/2015/11/29/opinion/sunday/contaminating-our-bodies-with-everyday-products.html.

18. For a detailed discussion of folate, the B vitamins and CoQ10, see Rebecca Fett, *It Starts with the Egg* (New York: Franklin Fox, 2016), 101–12.

19. I. M. Ebish, C. M. Thomas, W. H. Peters, et al., "The importance of Folate, Zinc and Antioxidants in the Pathogenesis and Prevention of Subfertility," *Human Reproduction Update* 12, no. 2 (March–April): 163–74.

20. See, for example, A. J. Gaskins, S. L. Mumford, J. E. Chavarro, et al., "The Impact of Dietary Folate Intake on Reproductive Function in Premenopausal Women: A Prospective Cohort Study," K. A. O'Connor, ed. *PLoS ONE* 7, no. 9 (2012): e46276; I. Dudás, M. Rockenbauer, and A. E. Czeizel, "The Effect of Preconceptional Multivitamin Supplementation on the Menstrual Cycle," *Archives of Gynecology and Obstetrics* 256, no. 3 (1995): 115.

21. J. C. Boxmeer, R. M. Brounds, J. Lindemans, et al., "Preconception Folic Acid Treatment Affects the Microenvironment of the Maturing Oocyte in Humans," *Fertility and Sterility* 89, no. 6 (June 2008):1766–70.

22. A. Turi, S. R. Giannubilo, F. Brugè, et al., "Coenzyme Q10 Content in Follicular Fluid and Its Relationship with Oocyte Fertilization and Embryo Grading," *Archives of Gynecology and Obstetrics* 285, no. 4 (April 2012): 1173–76.

23. J. Van Blerkom, "Mitochondrial Function in the Human Oocyte and Embryo and Their Role in Developmental Competence," *Mitochondrion* 11, no. 5 (September 2011): 797–813.

24. Y. Bentov, N. Esfandiari, E. Burstein, and R. F. Casper, "The Use of Mitochondrial Nutrients to Improve the Outcome of Infertility Treatment in Older Patients," *Fertility and Sterility* 93, no. 1 (January 2010): 272–75; A. Ben-Meir, E. Burstein, A. Borrego-Alvarez, et al., "Coenzyme Q10

Restores Oocyte Mitochondrial Function and Fertility During Reproductive Aging," *Aging Cell* 14, no. 5 (October 2015): 887–95.

25. M. Susiarjo, T. J. Hassold, E. Freeman, and P. A. Hunt, "Bisphenol A Exposure In Utero Disrupts Early Oogenesis in the Mouse," *PLoS Genetics* 3, no. 1 (January 2007): e5; P. Allard and M. P. Colaiácovo, "Bisphenol A Impairs the Double-Strand Break Repair Machinery in the Germline and Causes Chromosome Abnormalities," *Proceedings of the National Academy of Sciences* 107, no. 47 (November 23, 2010): 20405–10; J. Peretz, R. K. Gupta, J. Singh, et al., "Bisphenol A Impairs Follicle Growth, Inhibits Steroidogenesis, and Downregulates Rate-Limiting Enzymes in the Estradiol Biosynthesis Pathway," *Toxicological Sciences* 119, no. 1 (January 2011): 209–17.

26. V. Y. Fujimoto, D. Kim, F. S. vom Saal, et al., "Serum Unconjugated Bisphenol A Concentrations in Women May Adversely Influence Oocyte Quality During In Vitro Fertilization," *Fertility and Sterility*, 95, no. 5 (April 2011): 1816–19.

27. S. R. Ehrlich, P. L. Williams, S. A. Missmer, et al., "Urinary Bisphenol A Concentrations and Implantation Failure among Women Undergoing *In Vitro* Fertilization," *Fertility and Sterility* 92, no. 3, supplement (September 2009): S136.

28. M. S. Bloom, D. Kim, F. S. Vom Saal, et al., "Bisphenol A Exposure Reduces the Estradiol Response to Gonadotropin Stimulation During In Vitro Fertilization," *Fertility and Sterility* 96, no. 3 (September 2011): 672–77.e2; E. Mok-Lin, S. Ehrlich, P. L. Williams, et al., "Urinary Bisphenol A Concentrations and Ovarian Response Among Women Undergoing IVF," *International Journal of Andrology* 33, no. 2 (April 2010): 385–93.

29. R. B. Lathi, C. A. Liebert, K. F. Brookfield, et al., "Conjugated Bisphenol A in Maternal Serum in Relation to Miscarriage Risk," *Fertility and Sterility* 102, no. 1 (July 2014):123–28.

30. M. Sugiura-Ogasawara, Y. Ozaki, S. Sonta, et al., "Exposure to Bisphenol A Is Associated with Recurrent Miscarriage," *Human Reproduction* 20, no. 8 (August 2005): 2325–29.

31. Nagaoka et al., "Human Aneuploidy," 502.

32. Roger Highfield, "IVF Success Rate Is Too Low, Says Lord Winston," *The Telegraph,* June 9, 2008, http://www.telegraph.co.uk/news/science/science-news/3343919/IVF-success-rate-is-too-low-says-Lord-Winston.html.

33. Bart C. J. M. Fauser, "Relevance of embryo competence for successful IVF,

and role of GCSF," presentation at the 24th World Congress on Controversies in Obstetrics, Gynecology & Infertility (COGI), Amsterdam, November 11, 2016.

34. M. A. Santos, E. W. Kuijk, and N. S. Macklon, "The Impact of Ovarian Stimulation for IVF on the Developing Embryo," *Reproduction* 139, no. 1 (January 2010): 23–34.

35. Jacques Cohen, "MRT and PGD As a First-Line Treatment for Mitochondrial Disorders," presentation at the 24th World Congress on Controversies in Obstetrics, Gynecology & Infertility (COGI), November 12, 2016.

36. M. F. Verberg, M. J. Eijkemans, N. S. Macklon, et al., "The Clinical Significance of the Retrieval of a Low Number of Oocytes Following Mild Ovarian Stimulation for IVF: A Meta-analysis," *Human Reproduction Update* 15, no. 1 (January-February 2009): 5–12.

37. Rubio et al., "Prospective Cohort Study."

38. Grabar and Stefanovich, "Aneuploidies in Oocytes Used."

39. G. N. Allahbadia, "Have We Finally Written the Obituary for Conventional IVF?," *IVF Lite* 1, no. 1 (2014): 1–5.

40. J. J. Zhang, Z. Merhi, M. Yang, et al., "Minimal Stimulation IVF versus Conventional IVF: A Randomized Controlled Trial," *American Journal of Obstetrics & Gynecology* 214, no. 1 (January 2016): 96.e1–8.

41. Kato, "Natural-Cycle IVF" presentation.

42. Dr. Bernstein served as a lead investigator in these studies, using humanlike models of midlife female mice. She performed initial studies with Professor Duane Kraemer and colleagues at Texas A&M University, then with University of Maryland School of Medicine professors Istvan Merchenthaler and Charles Chaffin, and research assistant Amelia Mackenzie. See L. R. Bernstein, A. C. Mackenzie, S. J. Lee, et al., "Activin Decoy Receptor ActRIIB:Fc Lowers FSH and Therapeutically Restores Oocyte Yield, Prevents Oocyte Chromosome Misalignments and Spindle Aberrations, and Increases Fertility in Midlife Female SAMP8 Mice," *Endocrinology* 157, no. 3 (March 2016): 1234–47.

43. Pregmama, "About," http://www.datlof.com/2Pregmama/about.cfm.

44. Lori R. Bernstein, "Hormone Normalization Therapy Comprising Administration of Aromatase Inhibitor, Follicle Stimulating Hormone, Luteinizing Hormone, Human Chorionic Gonadotropin, Gonadotropin Hormone Releasing Hormone and/or Progesterone," US Patent application No. US9,056,072 B2, filed June 16, 2015.

Chapter 14

1. Fertility Authority, "New York Infertility Insurance Mandate," accessed December 11, 2017, https://www.fertilityauthority.com/costs/insurance-coverage/new-york-infertility-insurance-mandate. New York Consolidated Laws, Insurance, Sections 3221 and 4303.

2. See Infertility Resources, "Pharmacies," http://www.ihr.com/infertility/provider/pharmacy.html, for a list of domestic and international pharmacies.

3. What to Expect, "Fertility Treatments—Jobs with Infertility Coverage," accessed December 11, 2017, http://www.whattoexpect.com/forums/fertility-treatments/topic/jobs-with-infertility-coverage-51.html.

4. Laura Lorenzetti, "These 11 Companies Offer 100% Healthcare Coverage," *Fortune*, March 11, 2015, http://fortune.com/2015/03/11/companies-offer-all-healthcare-coverage/.

5. FertilityIQ, "The FertilityIQ Family Builder Workplace Index: 2017–2018," accessed December 10, 2017, https://www.fertilityiq.com/fertilityiq-data-and-notes/fertilityiq-best-companies-to-work-for-family-builder-workplace-index-2017-2018.

6. Shelby Livingston, "Fertility Treatment Costs Scare Off Employers," *Business Insurance*, January 17, 2016, http://www.businessinsurance.com/article/20160117/NEWS03/160119856/fertility-treatment-costs-scare-off-employers-but-those-who-offer.

7. Anna Medaris Miller, "Should You Travel Abroad for IVF?," *U.S. News & World Report*, December 15, 2015; Fertility Treatment Abroad, "IVF Prices: What Is the Cost of Fertility Treatment Abroad?," accessed December 11, 2017, http://fertility.treatmentabroad.com/costs. See also www.patientsbeyondborders.com.

8. Robert Winston, "Robert Winston: 'I Do Have a Very Dark Side,'" *The Telegraph*, August 15, 2008, http://www.telegraph.co.uk/news/features/3637695/Robert-WinstonI-do-have-a-very-dark-side.html.

9. FertilityIQ, "About us," accessed March 1, 2018, https://www.fertilityiq.com/who-we-are.

10. FertilityIQ, "FertilityIQ Data & Notes," accessed December 11, 2017, https://www.fertilityiq.com/fertilityiq-data-and-notes.

11. Tamar Lewin, "Industry's Growth Leads to Leftover Embryos, and

Painful Choices," *New York Times*, June 17, 2015, https://www.nytimes.com /2015/06/18/us/embryos-egg-donors-difficult-issues.html?_r=0.

12. Nick Loeb, "Sofía Vergara's Ex-Fiancé: Our Frozen Embryos Have a Right to Live," *New York Times*, April 29, 2015, https://www.nytimes.com /2015/04/30/opinion/sofiavergaras-ex-fiance-our-frozen-embryos -have-a-right-to-live.html.

13. Reber v. Reiss, 42 A.3d 1131 (Pa. Super. Ct. 2012); Angie Leventis Lourgos, "Judge Gives Embryos to Woman Over Objection from Ex-boyfriend," *Chicago Tribune*, May 16, 2014, http://www.chicagotribune.com/news /local/breaking/chi-judge-gives-embryos-to-woman-over-objection -from-exboyfriend-20140516-story.html.

14. The eight states that permit embryonic stem cell research as of 2016 are California, Connecticut, Illinois, Iowa, Maryland, Massachusetts, New Jersey, and New York. States that restrict or ban it include Florida, Indiana, Kentucky, North Dakota, Ohio, Oklahoma, and South Dakota. For a complete list, see National Conference of State Legislatures, "Embryonic and Fetal Research Laws," January 1, 2016, http://www.ncsl.org/research /health/embryonic-and-fetal-research-laws.aspx.

15. Andrew Vorzimer, "Get Pregnant with Built-On Spec Embryos or Get Your Money Back!," *The Spin Doctor*, http://www.eggdonor.com/blog /2012/11/20/pregnant-built-spec-embryos-money/.

16. Lewin, "Industry's Growth."

17. Stein, "New York Fertility Doctor."

18. Charlotte Pritchard, "The Girl with Three Biological Parents," *BBC News Magazine*, September 1, 2014, http://www.bbc.com/news/magazine -28986843.

19. Conor Gaffey, "Three-Person Baby Born in Ukraine After Doctors Use Novel Technique," *Newsweek*, January 18, 2017, http://www.newsweek.com/three -person-baby-born-ukraine-after-doctors-use-novel-technique-543878.

20. The CRISPR-Cas9 is a two-part molecular scissors comprising a DNA-cutting protein called Cas9 and a short piece of RNA that guides the protein to a gene that scientists want to snip.

21. T. H. Saey, "New Era of Human Embryo Gene Editing Begins," *Science News* 190, no. 9 (October 29, 2016): 15. See also E. Callaway, "Gene-editing Research in Human Embryos Gains Momentum," *Nature* 532, no. 7,599 (April 21, 2016): 289–90.

22. Myers et al., "Effectiveness of Assisted Reproductive Technology (ART)."

23. Eliza Barclay, "Scientists Successfully Used CRISPR to Fix a Mutation That Causes Disease. This Is Huge," *Vox*, August 2, 2017, https://www.vox.com/science-and-health/2017/8/2/16083300/crispr-heart-disease.

Index

About the Author

ELIZABETH KATKIN, a lawyer and mother of two, is a former partner at a large international law firm. A graduate of Yale College and Columbia University's Law School and School of International and Public Affairs, she lives with her husband, Richard, and their children in Denver, Colorado. *Conceivability* is her first book.